DRUG DOSAGES AND SOLUTIONS:
A WORKBOOK

Second Edition

DRUG DOSAGES AND SOLUTIONS: A WORKBOOK

Second Edition

Mary Ann Fravel Norville R.N., B.S.N., M.Ed.
Assistant Professor
Essex Community College
Baltimore, Maryland

APPLETON & LANGE
Norwalk, Connecticut/San Mateo, California

0-8385-1740-4

Copyright © 1988, 1982 by Mary Ann Fravel Norville
Published by Appleton & Lange
A Publishing Division of Prentice Hall

88 89 90 91 92 / 10 9 8 7 6 5 4 3 2 1

Prentice-Hall of Australia, Pty, Ltd., Sydney
Prentice-Hall Canada, Inc.
Prentice-Hall Hispanoamericana, S.A., Mexico
Prentice-Hall of India Private Limited, New Delhi
Prentice-Hall International (UK) Limited, London
Prentice-Hall of Japan, Inc., Tokyo
Prentice-Hall of Southeast Asia (Pte.) Ltd., Singapore
Whitehall Books Ltd., Wellington, New Zealand
Editora Prentice-Hall do Brasil Ltda., Rio de Janeiro

Library of Congress Cataloging-in-Publication Data

Norville, Mary Ann Fravel.
   Drug dosages and solutions: a workbook / Mary Ann Fravel
Norville.—2nd ed.
     p. cm.
   Rev. ed. of: Drug dosages and solutions workbook. ©1982.
   ISBN 0-8385-1740-4
   1. Pharmaceutical arithmetic. 2. Drugs—Dosage. 3. Solutions
(Pharmacy) 4. Nursing—Mathematics. I. Norville, Mary Ann Fravel.
Drug dosages and solutions workbook. II. Title.
   [DNLM: 1. Drugs—administration & dosage—problems.
2. Mathematics—problems. 3. Solutions—administration & dosage—
problems. QV 18 N891d]
RS57.N67 1988   87-31937
615′.14′076—dc19   CIP

Production Editor: Charles F. Evans
Designer: Kathleen Peters Ceconi

PRINTED IN THE UNITED STATES OF AMERICA

To my husband, Charles.

Contents

Preface

In offering this second edition of my textbook to my colleagues and students, I wish to reaffirm my purposes as stated in the original edition, which were to facilitate the learning of dosage by nursing students (and by others in the health care professions) by presenting dosage in a manner that was clear and concise, and in a way in which the principles and problems of dosages and solutions might be simply stated, without compromising either the necessary information, or insulting the intelligence of the student. The acceptance of my original work by so many of my professional colleagues and their many favorable comments confirm my belief that such a text is needed, and justify the preparation of a second, enlarged edition.

Many new dosage problems have been added throughout the book, and I demonstrate how each problem can be solved by using either the ratio–proportion or the formula method. Practice problems have been included after each new explanation. The chapters have been rearranged so that problems based on the metric system are placed first. Recognizing a growing trend toward home health care, I have discussed household units of measurement and conversions from the metric system to make it easier for professionals to instruct clients in self-medication. The chapter on solutions has been clarified with explanations and practice problems using examples of solutions that might be used in home health situations.

Several chapters have been considerably enlarged, especially the chapters dealing with pediatrics and intravenous fluids, insulin, and solutions. In the chapter on pediatric dosage I have emphasized the need to confirm the appropriate dosage for an infant or child, and I have clarified and added new problems emphasizing dose per weight. The explanations have been rewritten for body surface area and nomogram use. I have de-emphasized Clark's, Fried's, and Young's rules, but include them for the benefit of those who may desire to use them.

The chapter on intravenous fluid rate calculations has been expanded. I use a simple two-step method to compute the large-volume IV flow rate. Only the second step is used to compute the flow rate for small-volume IVs, thus reducing the number of different formulas to be memorized. The section on flow rate calculation for large-volume IVs, how to deliver an ordered amount of drug per hour or per minute, has been expanded. Two new sections explain calculations for volume control sets (i.e., the Buretrol), how to determine if an IV is running off schedule, and how to correct this problem. All sections in the chapter contain practice problems.

The chapter on insulin includes the use of both an insulin syringe and cubic centimeter syringe.

Drug labels, syringes, and medicine cups are depicted throughout the text to make the problems more realistic for the student. I have included a new chapter on how to read the calibrations on the five syringes most frequently used to administer parenteral medications. I have also included a table of abbreviations commonly used in administering medications. This appears in the book's inside front cover for easy student reference.

Throughout, in revising the text, I have paid close attention to the criticism and suggestions of my colleagues and my students, rewriting and expanding areas in the original edition that were not clear to them. I thank my colleagues and my students for their thoughtful comments and suggestions.

Acknowledgments

I express my sincere appreciation to the many persons and drug companies who have helped me to complete this second edition of my book.

To my husband, Charles, who patiently read and critiqued my manuscript; to my family, for prodding me and encouraging me until this revision was completed.

To Jeffrey Longcope, former Nursing Editor of Appleton & Lange Publishers, for his advice, encouragement and support; to Joanne Jay, Director, Art/Editorial Production, for her many helpful suggestions; to Charles Evans, Production Editor, for his help and guidance through the editing process; and to all others at Appleton & Lange who have helped with the production of the second edition of this textbook.

To William L. Robinson, Jr., graphic artist, Essex Community College, my grateful appreciation for his graphic art work depicting the volume control set and syringes; to Carolyn Insley, who typed most of the manuscript and related correspondence, a special word of thanks for her friendship, patience, and understanding throughout; to Ruth Wright, and to Charles and Valerie Norville, who assisted with the typing.

To Helen V. Kramer, Professor of Nursing Emerita at Essex Community College, for her support from when I first discussed this book to the present; to my nursing faculty colleagues at Essex Community College, especially Terry Bianco and Karen Cooper who advised me about pediatric dosages, and Terry Majewski for her positive evaluation of my textbook; to my former colleague, Barbara Wise, who read and critiqued the pediatric chapter. In addition, I am grateful to my colleagues in the Allied Health and Mathematics Divisions of Essex Community College for their relevant insights and suggestions.

To Dr. Thomas M. Holcomb, Chairman of the Department of Pediatrics, and to the pharmacists and the many nurses at The Franklin Square Hospital, who helped and advised me on possible dosage problems; to Dr. Billy Wickcliffe, Assistant Professor of Pharmacy, University of Georgia, School of Pharmacy for her patience and wise counsel; to Mary Ann Hardage, Staff Pharmacist, St. Mary's Hospital, Athens, Georgia, for her help.

To the following pharmaceutical companies for the use of their copyrighted drug labels and/or pictures of equipment: Abbott Laboratories; Ivac Corporation; Eli Lilly & Company; Elkins-Sinn, Inc., a subsidiary of A. H. Robins Company; Merck, Sharp & Dohme, Division of Merck and Company; Parke Davis, Division of Warner-Lambert Company; Pfizer Laboratories Division; Roerig, a Division of Pfizer Pharmaceuticals; Smith Kline and French Laboratories, a Smith Kline Beckman Company; and to all of the others who extended their courtesy and help to me.

Also, printed with permission by Bristol-Myers U.S. Pharmaceutical and Nutritional Group into the second edition of this textbook, the following drug labels: Dynapen 62.5 mg/5 ml; Polycillin 500 mg capsules; Polycillin-N 1 g for IM or IV use; Prostaphlin 500 mg for injection; Cefadyl 1 g for IV use; Amikin (Amikacin Sulfate injection) 500 mg/2 ml; Amikin (Amikacin Sulfate) 100 mg/2 ml; Polymox 125 mg/bottle; Cefadyl 1 g IV.

And, last but not least, I express my appreciation to my students (both past and present) for whom this book is written. Their words of praise and gratitude to me, along with their many helpful criticisms and suggestions, have made, and continue to make this project so worthwhile.

Introduction to Dosage and Solutions

In 1975 Congress passed the Metric Conversion Act, which states that the United States will convert to the metric system of weights and measures at some indefinite time in the future. We see some evidence of conversion to the metric system, for example, bottling companies are supplying soft drinks in metric measures, gasoline is being sold by the liter, and highway mileage signs are being posted in kilometers. In addition, modern measuring cups are inscribed with both metric and household measures.

In medicine, too, the trend has been toward the metric system. All drugs are now manufactured in metric units. Some drugs that have been used for many years also carry the apothecaries' equivalent on the label. Physicians trained in apothecaries' units still order drugs by this system of measurement. Therefore, nurses must know both the metric and the apothecaries' system to safely administer medications. In a recent survey of the hospitals and nursing homes in the state of Maryland, and in some other states as well, I found that the apothecaries' system is still being used by some physicians to order drugs.

In addition to these two systems, the nurse must be familiar with the household system used to teach self-medication in the home. Each of these three systems has different symbols and abbreviations. *Conversions among the three systems are only approximate; there are no absolute equivalents among the systems.* Each of these systems of measurement is discussed separately in the following chapters. First, I discuss the metric system, and explain how to solve problems using this system. The apothecaries' system and the household system are discussed afterward, along with methods of converting equivalent values from one system to the other.

DRUG DOSAGES AND SOLUTIONS: A WORKBOOK

Second Edition

Arithmetic Self-evaluation

To begin your study of dosage and solutions, first review your basic math skills by doing this self-evaluation.

The number concepts needed to master the content of this dosage workbook are exemplified in the following problems. Work each set of examples to see if you remember how to find the answer. The explanations and answers are found on the pages following the test.

1. *Circle the largest number in each set. Underline the smallest number.*

   a. $\dfrac{1}{4}, \dfrac{4}{8}, \dfrac{3}{16}$

   b. $\dfrac{8}{9}, \dfrac{8}{25}, \dfrac{8}{125}$

   c. 0.5, 0.25, 0.125

   d. 0.325, 1.3333, 1.75

2. *Add the following fractions and mixed numbers.*

   a. $\dfrac{7}{8} + \dfrac{5}{4} = $ _____

   b. $10\dfrac{1}{2} + 12\dfrac{1}{4} + 16\dfrac{3}{4} = $ _____

   c. $\dfrac{3}{4} + \dfrac{1}{6} + \dfrac{1}{8} = $ _____

d. $7\dfrac{1}{12} + 3\dfrac{2}{3} + 8\dfrac{5}{24} =$ _____

3. *Add the following decimals.*

    a. $10.4 + 45.62 + 0.44 =$ _____

    b. $0.01 + 0.625 + 2.3 =$ _____

    c. $16 + 8.24 + 0.084 =$ _____

    d. $0.125 + 0.025 + 0.05 =$ _____

4. *Subtract the following fractions and mixed numbers.*

    a. $\dfrac{2}{3} - \dfrac{1}{4} =$ _____

    b. $6\dfrac{2}{5} - 5\dfrac{3}{10} =$ _____

    c. $100\dfrac{1}{33} - 33\dfrac{1}{3} =$ _____

    d. $175\dfrac{4}{6} - 148\dfrac{1}{3} =$ _____

5. *Subtract the following decimal fractions.*

    a. $950 - 250.25 =$ _____

    b. $0.05 - 0.025 =$ _____

    c. $16.23 - 14.293 =$ _____

    d. $2.8 - 0.95 =$ _____

6. *Multiply the following fractions.*

    a. $\dfrac{2}{4} \times \dfrac{4}{6} =$ _____

    b. $\dfrac{1}{2} \times \dfrac{1}{3} =$ _____

    c. $5\dfrac{1}{6} \times \dfrac{1}{8} =$ _____

    d. $4\dfrac{4}{5} \times 2\dfrac{1}{5} \times 8\dfrac{1}{4} =$ _____

7. *Multiply the following decimals.*

    a. $1.5 \times 3 =$ _____

    b. $0.05 \times 1.5 =$ _____

    c. $36.284 \times 7.21 =$ _____

    d. $0.0033 \times 6.02 =$ _____

8. *Divide the following fractions.*

    a. $\dfrac{1}{2} \div \dfrac{1}{3} =$ _____

    b. $\dfrac{1}{150} \div \dfrac{1}{2} =$ _____

    c. $3\dfrac{3}{4} \div \dfrac{2}{3} =$ _____

    d. $\dfrac{1\frac{1}{2}}{\frac{7}{8}} \div \dfrac{1\frac{1}{3}}{2\frac{1}{2}} =$ _____

9. *Divide the following decimals.*

    a. $64.5 \div 2.5 =$ _____

    b. $2.5 \div 0.01 =$ _____

    c. $12.075 \div 2.5 =$ _____

    d. $0.065 \div 10 =$ _____

10. *Solve for* N *using a formula and prove your answer.*

    a. $\dfrac{24}{48} \times 5 = N$

    b. $\dfrac{120}{60} \times 2.2 = N$

    c. $\dfrac{3.5}{1.75} \times 5 = N$

    d. $\dfrac{32}{16} \times N = 60$

    e. $\dfrac{4}{9} \times N = 8$

f. $\dfrac{N}{4} \times 6 = 4.5$

g. $\dfrac{N}{8} \times 4 = 3$

h. $\dfrac{6}{N} \times 6 = 4$

11. *Solve for* x *using the ratio–proportion method and prove your answer.*

   a. $5:20::2:x$

   b. $\dfrac{1}{6}:1::x:1\dfrac{1}{2}$

   c. $\dfrac{2.5}{x} :: \dfrac{5}{10}$

   d. $\dfrac{x}{\frac{3}{4}} :: \dfrac{\frac{7}{9}}{\frac{21}{24}}$

   e. $x:16::4:8$

   f. $27:x::9:3$

   g. $\dfrac{4}{5} :: \dfrac{20}{x}$

   h. $\dfrac{7}{8} :: \dfrac{x}{64}$

12. *Write the following Arabic numerals as Roman numerals.*

   a. 8 _____

   b. 3 _____

   c. 21 _____

   d. 50 _____

   e. 5 _____

   f. 14 _____

   g. 101 _____

   h. 1988 _____

13. *Write the following Roman numerals as Arabic numerals.*

    a. CIV _____

    b. XL _____

    c. MCMLXXXI _____

    d. XV _____

    e. IV _____

    f. XI _____

    g. XXXIV _____

    h. VII _____

14. *Convert the following units to the indicated equivalents.*

	Percentage	Decimal	Fraction	Ratio
a.	10%			
b.		0.65		
c.			$\frac{1}{4}$	
d.				1:500

15. *Round the following numbers as indicated.*

	Number	Round to the Nearest Whole Number	Round to the Nearest Tenth
a.	3.471		
b.	8.94		
c.	0.93		
d.	0.082		
e.	25.69		

	Number	Round to the Nearest Hundredth	Round to the Nearest Thousandth
f.	21.6107		
g.	4.2187		
h.	0.6709		
i.	8.4653		
j.	10.0294		

ANSWERS: ARITHMETIC SELF-EVALUATION

1. *Circle the largest number in each set. Underline the smallest number.*

    a. $\dfrac{1}{4}$, $\boxed{\dfrac{4}{8}}$, $\dfrac{3}{16}$

        $\dfrac{4}{16}$ $\dfrac{8}{16}$ $\dfrac{3}{16}$

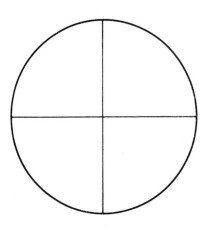

To compare the relative value of each fraction, first find the lowest common denominator for the group of fractions and then compare their value. To help you visualize these concepts, you might also think of these fractions in terms of familiar illustrations from life, for example, as the parts into which three pies are divided. You know that if you are served ¼ of a pie, the pie has been divided into four parts.

$\dfrac{1}{4}$ The *numerator* tells us how many parts are involved. The *denominator* tells us how many parts are in the whole (in this case, the number of parts into which the pie was divided) and the numerator tells you how many parts you received.

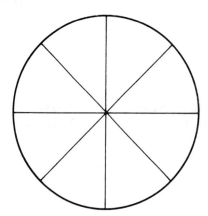

If the same pie were divided into eight parts, you know each part will be smaller, or ½ the size of those in the first pie. Since you will receive ⁴⁄₈ of the pie, you will receive 4 parts of the pie, which will equal ½ of the pie: ⁴⁄₈ = ½.

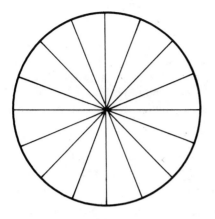

Now if the pie were divided into 16 parts, each part will be only a quarter of the size of those in the first pie. The three parts that you receive do not equal ¼ of the pie, as in the case of the pie divided into only four parts. You know that this is a smaller fraction.

b. numerator $\quad \left(\dfrac{8}{9}\right), \dfrac{8}{25}, \dfrac{8}{125}$
   denominator

The smaller the denominator, the greater the number of parts into which the whole has been divided. The larger the denominator, the smaller the number of parts into which the whole has been divided. The numerators are all the same. In the first fraction, 8/9, you are dealing with 8 parts out of a total of 9 parts. The second fraction is 8 parts out of a total of 25 parts. The third fraction is 8 parts out of a total of 125 parts—a much smaller proportion.

c. $\left(0.5\right)$, 0.25, 0.125

You may think of decimal fractions as 5/10, 25/100, and 125/1000.

$$\dfrac{5}{10} = \dfrac{1}{2} \qquad \dfrac{25}{100} = \dfrac{1}{4} \qquad \dfrac{125}{1000} = \dfrac{1}{8}$$

Another familiar example may involve money. 0.5 is the same as 0.50 or 50¢. 0.25 or 25¢ and 0.125 or 12½¢.

d.   0.325,   1.3333, $\left(1.75\right)$

Think fractions $\qquad \dfrac{325}{1000}, \quad 1\dfrac{3333}{10,000}, \quad 1\dfrac{75}{100}$

Numbers to the left of a decimal point are whole numbers.

or

Think money $\qquad 32\dfrac{1}{2}¢, \quad \$1.33\dfrac{1}{3}, \quad \$1.75$

Numbers to the right of a decimal point are fractions of a whole number.

2. *Add the following fractions and mixed numbers.*

a. numerator $\dfrac{7}{8}$ denominator $+ \dfrac{5}{4} = \dfrac{7}{8} + \dfrac{10}{8} = \dfrac{17}{8} = 2\dfrac{1}{8}$

When adding fractions you must *first* be sure that each fraction has the same denominator. If the denominators are not the same, find a common denominator. (A common denominator is a number into which all of the denominators will divide evenly.) *Next*, you must add the numerators together. In this example, you want to know how many 8ths you have. When added, you have 17 eighths. Divide 17 by 8 to change the fraction to a mixed number: $^{17}/_{8} = 2^{1}/_{8}$.

b.
$$10\dfrac{1}{2} = 10\dfrac{2}{4}$$
$$12\dfrac{1}{4} = 12\dfrac{1}{4}$$
$$16\dfrac{3}{4} = 16\dfrac{3}{4}$$
$$38\dfrac{6}{4} = 38 + 1\dfrac{2}{4}$$
$$= 38 + 1\dfrac{1}{2}$$
$$= 39\dfrac{1}{2}$$

Find a common denominator for the fractions and add the numerators to see how many 4ths you have. Add the whole numbers (10 + 12 + 16 = 38) and then add the fractions ($^{2}/_{4}$ + $^{1}/_{4}$ + $^{3}/_{4}$ = $^{6}/_{4}$). Reduce the improper fraction $^{6}/_{4}$ to $1^{1}/_{2}$ and add this to the sum of the whole numbers.

c. $\dfrac{3}{4} = \dfrac{18}{24}$

$\dfrac{1}{6} = \dfrac{4}{24}$

$\dfrac{1}{8} = \dfrac{3}{24}$

$\dfrac{25}{24} = 1\dfrac{1}{24}$

The least common denominator for 4, 6, and 8 is 24.

d. $7\dfrac{1}{12} = 7\dfrac{2}{24}$

$3\dfrac{2}{3} = 3\dfrac{16}{24}$

$8\dfrac{5}{24} = 8\dfrac{5}{24}$

$18\dfrac{23}{24}$

3. *Add the following decimals.*

a.
$$
\begin{array}{r}
10.40 \\
45.62 \\
0.44 \\
\hline
56.46
\end{array}
$$

You may add a zero to keep the columns straight. Line up the numbers so the decimal points are in a straight line. Then add the columns as you would whole numbers. Remember to place the decimal point in the answer. It should be placed directly under the other decimal points.

b.
$$
\begin{array}{r}
0.010 \\
0.625 \\
2.300 \\
\hline
2.935
\end{array}
$$

c.
$$
\begin{array}{r}
16.000 \\
8.240 \\
0.084 \\
\hline
24.324
\end{array}
$$

d.
$$
\begin{array}{r}
0.125 \\
0.025 \\
0.050 \\
\hline
0.200
\end{array}
$$

4. *Subtract the following fractions and mixed numbers.*

a.
$$
\begin{array}{rcr}
\dfrac{2}{3} & = & \dfrac{8}{12} \\[2ex]
-\dfrac{1}{4} & = & -\dfrac{3}{12} \\[2ex]
\hline
& & \dfrac{5}{12}
\end{array}
$$

Before you can subtract fractions you must find a common denominator.

b.
$$
\begin{array}{rcr}
6\dfrac{2}{5} & = & 6\dfrac{4}{10} \\[2ex]
-5\dfrac{3}{10} & = & -5\dfrac{3}{10} \\[2ex]
\hline
& & 1\dfrac{1}{10}
\end{array}
$$

c.
$$
100\dfrac{1}{33} = \dfrac{99}{\cancel{100}} \dfrac{+1}{33} = 99\dfrac{34}{33}
$$
$$
-33\dfrac{1}{3} = -33\dfrac{11}{33} = -33\dfrac{11}{33}
$$
$$
\overline{\qquad\qquad\qquad 66\dfrac{23}{33}}
$$

In this problem, you cannot subtract ¹¹⁄₃₃ from ¹⁄₃₃, so you must borrow 1 or ³³⁄₃₃ from 100, add it to ¹⁄₃₃, giving you ³⁴⁄₃₃.

Next, subtract as in the other problems.

d.
$$
\begin{array}{rcr}
175\dfrac{4}{6} & = & 175\dfrac{4}{6} \\[2ex]
-148\dfrac{1}{3} & = & -148\dfrac{2}{6} \\[2ex]
\hline
& & 27\dfrac{2}{6} = 27\dfrac{1}{3}
\end{array}
$$

5. *Subtract the following decimal fractions.*

<table>
<tr><td>a.</td><td>950.00
−250.25
─────
699.75</td><td>Line up the decimal points and numbers in straight lines and then proceed as with whole numbers.</td></tr>
</table>

Remember to bring the decimal point down.

<table>
<tr><td>b.</td><td>0.050
−0.025
─────
0.025</td><td>A zero to the left of the decimal indicates there is no whole number. The number is less than 1.</td></tr>
</table>

c. 16.230
  −14.293
  ─────
   1.937

d. 2.80
  −0.95
  ─────
   1.85

6. *Multiply the following fractions.*

a. $\dfrac{2}{4} \times \dfrac{4}{6} = \dfrac{8}{24} = \dfrac{1}{3}$

(1) Multiply the numerators and denominators. It is not necessary to find a common denominator. (2) When multiplying or dividing fractions, reduce the fractions to the lowest term.

b. $\dfrac{1}{2} \times \dfrac{1}{3} = \dfrac{1}{6}$

c. $5\dfrac{1}{6} \times \dfrac{1}{8} = \dfrac{31}{6} \times \dfrac{1}{8} = \dfrac{31}{48}$

Mixed numbers, i.e., 5⅙, must be changed to improper fractions. Multiply the whole number by the denominator and add to the numerator. Multiply the numerators and the denominators.

d. $4\dfrac{4}{5} \times 2\dfrac{1}{5} \times 8\dfrac{1}{4} = \dfrac{24}{5} \times \dfrac{11}{5} \times \dfrac{33}{4} = \dfrac{8712}{100} = 87\dfrac{12}{100} = 87\dfrac{3}{25}$

7. *Multiply the following decimals.*

a. 1.5   multiplicand
  ×3   multiplier
 ─────
  4.5   product

Multiply decimal fractions as you would multiply whole numbers. To determine where to place the decimal point in the product, count the number of places to the right of the decimal in both the multiplicand and the multi-plier. The number of decimal places in the product is equal to the sum of the decimal places in the multiplicand and the multiplier.

b.
$$
\begin{array}{r}
0.05 \\
\times 1.5 \\
\hline
25 \\
5 \\
\hline
0.075
\end{array}
$$

c.
$$
\begin{array}{r}
36.284 \\
\times 7.21 \\
\hline
36284 \\
72568 \\
253988 \\
\hline
261.60764
\end{array}
$$

d.
$$
\begin{array}{r}
0.0033 \\
\times 6.02 \\
\hline
66 \\
0 \\
198 \\
\hline
0.019866
\end{array}
$$

8. *Divide the following fractions.*

Dividend Divisor

a. $\dfrac{1}{2} \div \dfrac{1}{3} = \dfrac{1}{2} \times \dfrac{3}{1} = \dfrac{3}{2} = 1\dfrac{1}{2}$

To divide fractions, invert the divisor (the number by which you are dividing) and then proceed as in mul-tiplication.

b. $\dfrac{1}{150} \div \dfrac{1}{2} =$

$\dfrac{1}{150} \times \dfrac{2}{1} = \dfrac{1}{75}$

c. $3\dfrac{3}{4} \div \dfrac{2}{3} =$

$\dfrac{15}{4} \times \dfrac{3}{2} = \dfrac{45}{8} = 5\dfrac{5}{8}$

Change the mixed number to an im-proper fraction and divide by inverting the divisor.

d. $\dfrac{1\frac{1}{2}}{\frac{7}{8}} \div \dfrac{1\frac{1}{3}}{2\frac{1}{2}} =$

$\dfrac{\frac{3}{2}}{\frac{7}{8}} \div \dfrac{\frac{4}{3}}{\frac{5}{2}} =$

$\dfrac{\frac{3}{2}}{\frac{7}{8}} \times \dfrac{\frac{5}{2}}{\frac{4}{3}} = \dfrac{\frac{15}{4}}{\frac{28}{24}} = \dfrac{15}{\cancel{4}} \times \dfrac{\cancel{24}^{6}}{28} = \dfrac{90}{28} = 3\dfrac{6}{28} = 3\dfrac{3}{14}$

Change the mixed numbers to im-proper fractions. Work with the prob-lem as if it contained whole numbers. Divide by inverting the ⁴⁄₃ over ⁵⁄₂ and multiply the fractions.

9. *Divide the following decimals and prove the answer.*

a.
$$64.5 \div 2.5 = \quad 2.5\overline{)64.5,0}$$
25.8 Quotient
Dividend
Divisor

Proof:
$$\begin{array}{r} 25.8 \\ \times 2.5 \\ \hline 1290 \\ 516 \\ \hline 64.50 \end{array}$$

To divide decimal fractions:
(1) Change the divisor to a whole number. To do this, move the decimal point enough places to the right to clear the decimal fraction. This is the same as multiplying the divisor by 10 or a multiple of 10. In the problem above, it is necessary to move the decimal point one place to the right or multiply by 10.

$$2.5 \times 10 = 25$$

(2) Use a caret (∧) to indicate the new position of the decimal point.
(3) Because you have moved the decimal point in the divisor to the right, you must multiply the dividend by 10, move the decimal point in the dividend an equal number of places to the right. Place a caret mark at the new location of the decimal point in the dividend.
(4) Divide the numbers.
(5) Place the decimal point in the quotient directly above the decimal point in the dividend. (See examples a, b, and c.)

b.
$$2.5 \div 0.01 = \quad 0.01\overline{)2.50,}$$
250.

Proof:
$$\begin{array}{r} 250 \\ \times 0.01 \\ \hline 2.50 \end{array}$$

c.
$$12.075 \div 2.5 = \quad 2.5\overline{)12.0,75}$$
4.83
$$\begin{array}{r} \underline{100} \\ 207 \\ \underline{200} \\ 75 \\ \underline{75} \\ 0 \end{array}$$

Proof:
$$\begin{array}{r} 4.83 \\ \times 2.5 \\ \hline 2415 \\ 966 \\ \hline 12.075 \end{array}$$

d.
$$0.065 \div 10 = 10\overline{)0.0650}\,^{0.0065}$$

Proof:
$$\begin{array}{r} 0.0065 \\ \times\,10 \\ \hline 0.0650 \end{array}$$

In this problem you cannot divide 10 into zero or into 6. Therefore, you must place zeros in the quotient after the decimal point to indicate that 10 would not divide into either number. It is *necessary in dosage to place a zero in front of the decimal point* to indicate that there is no whole number.

e.
$$250 \div 2.4 =$$

$$\begin{array}{r} 10\,4.16 \text{ r16} \\ 2.4\,\overline{)250.0\,00} \\ 24 \\ \hline 10 \\ 00 \\ \hline 100 \\ 96 \\ \hline 40 \\ 24 \\ \hline 160 \\ 144 \\ \hline 16 \end{array}$$

Proof:
$$\begin{array}{r} 104.16 \\ \times\,2.4 \\ \hline 41664 \\ 20832 \\ \hline 249.984 \\ +16\text{r} \\ \hline 250.000 \end{array}$$

One of the most common errors students make in dividing is failing to place a zero in the quotient when the divisor is greater than the number in the dividend. (For example, 24 will not divide into 10. Place a zero in the quotient and bring down the next number; 24 will divide into 100 four times.) Continue to divide to the hundredths place. There will be a remainder of 16. This problem will never divide to an even number.

 To prove the answer is correct, multiply the quotient by the divisor and add the remainder, 16, to this answer. The new answer should equal the number in the dividend.

f.
$$88 \div 2.2 = 2.2\,\overline{)88.0}\,^{4\,0.} \\ 88 \\ \overline{00}$$

$$= \quad \begin{array}{r} 40. \\ 22\overline{)880.} \\ 88 \\ \hline 00 \end{array}$$

Proof:
$$\begin{array}{r} 2.2 \\ \times\,40 \\ \hline 88.0 \end{array}$$

To remove the decimal in the divisor in this problem, move it one place to the right. In the dividend the decimal belongs after the 88. Put the decimal in its place and then move it one place to the right by adding a zero. Divide 880 by 22. Do not forget to place the zero after the 4. In the quotient, 880 divided by 22 equals 40, not just 4.

g.
$$16940 \div 0.28 =$$

$$0.28\overline{)16940.00}$$
605 00.
$$\underline{168}$$
14
$$\underline{00}$$
140
$$\underline{140}$$
0

Proof:
60500
$$\underline{\times 0.28}$$
484000
$$\underline{121000}$$
16940.00

h.
$$72.208 \div 8 =$$

$$8\overline{)72.208}$$
9.026
$$\underline{72}$$
002
$$\underline{000}$$
20
$$\underline{16}$$
48
$$\underline{48}$$
0

Proof:
9.026
$$\underline{\times 8}$$
72.208

10. *Solve for* N *using a formula.*

a. $\dfrac{24}{48} \times 5 = N$

Multiply the fraction in the usual manner to solve for *N*.

$$\dfrac{\overset{1}{\cancel{24}}}{\underset{6}{\cancel{48}}} \times \dfrac{5}{1} = \dfrac{15}{6} = 2\dfrac{1}{2}$$

b. $\dfrac{120}{60} \times 2.2 = N$

$$\dfrac{\overset{2}{\cancel{120}}}{\underset{1}{\cancel{60}}} \times \dfrac{2.2}{1} = 4.4$$

c. $\dfrac{3.5}{1.75} \times 5 = N$

$$\dfrac{3.5}{1.75} \times \dfrac{5}{1} = \dfrac{17.5}{1.75} = 10$$

Proof:

$$1.75\overline{)17.50}$$
10
$$\underline{175}$$
00

d. $\dfrac{32}{16} \times N = 60$

$$\dfrac{\overset{2}{\cancel{32}}}{\underset{1}{\cancel{16}}} \times N = 60$$

In this problem, the unknown factor is multiplied by the fraction. To find the value of *N*, divide both sides of the equation by $^{32}/_{16}$ (or $^{2}/_{1}$ if you prefer to reduce the fraction $^{32}/_{16} =$

$$\frac{2}{1} \div \frac{2}{1} \times N = 60 \div \frac{2}{1}$$

$$\frac{2}{1} \times \frac{1}{2} \times N = \overset{30}{\cancel{60}} \times \frac{1}{\cancel{2}_1} = 30$$

$$N = 30$$

²⁄₁). To check the equation, substitute 30 for N; multiply to see if the answer is 60.

Proof:

$$\frac{\overset{2}{\cancel{32}}}{\underset{1}{\cancel{16}}} \times 30 = 60$$

e. $$\frac{4}{9} \times N = 8$$

$$\frac{4}{9} \times \frac{9}{4} N = 8 \times \frac{9}{4}$$

$$N = \frac{72}{4}$$

$$N = 18$$

Proof:

$$\frac{4}{\cancel{9}_1} \times \overset{2}{\cancel{18}} = 8$$

f. $$\frac{N}{4} \times 6 = 4.5$$

$$\frac{6N}{4} \div \frac{6}{4} = 4.5 \div \frac{6}{4}$$

$$\frac{\cancel{6}N}{\cancel{4}} \times \frac{\cancel{4}}{\cancel{6}} = 4.5 \times \frac{4}{6} = \frac{18}{6}$$

$$N = 3$$

Proof:

$$\frac{3}{4} \times 6 = \frac{18}{4} = 4.5$$

g. $$\frac{N}{8} \times 4 = 3$$

$$\frac{4N}{8} \div \frac{4}{8} = 3 \div \frac{4}{8}$$

$$\frac{\cancel{4}N}{\cancel{8}} \times \frac{\cancel{8}}{\cancel{4}} = 3 \times \frac{8}{4} = \frac{24}{4}$$

$$N = 6$$

Proof:

$$\frac{6}{8} \times 4 = \frac{24}{8} = 3$$

h. $$\frac{6}{N} \times 6 = 4$$

$$\frac{36}{N} = 4$$

$$\frac{36}{N} \times \frac{N}{1} = 4 \times \frac{N}{1}$$

$$36 = 4N$$

$$\frac{36}{4} = \frac{4N}{4}$$

$$9 = N$$

Proof:

$$\frac{6}{9} \times 6 = \frac{36}{9} = 4$$

11. *Solve for* x *using the ratio–proportion method and prove your answers.*

a. A *proportion* consists of two ratios that have equivalent values. A *ratio* consists of two numbers separated by a colon, indicating a relationship exists between the two numbers.

$$5:20::2:x$$

means

extremes

$$5x = 40$$

$$\frac{5}{5}x = \frac{40}{5}$$

$$x = 8$$

OR

$$\frac{5}{20} \times \frac{2}{x}$$

$$5x = 40$$

$$\frac{5x}{5} = \frac{40}{5}$$

$$x = 8$$

To solve this problem, multiply the extremes (the two outside numbers) and then multiply the means (the two inside numbers). Solve for *x*. In a true proportion, the product of the means equals the product of the extremes. You may check your answer by substituting the value of *x* into the proportion, multiplying the means and then the extremes, confirming that they are equal. The two ratios in the proportion may be set up as fractions. Cross multiply. In order to be consistent, keep the unknown factor on the left side and the known factor on the right side of the equation.

Proof:

$$5:20::2:8$$

$$20 \times 2 = 5 \times 8$$

$$40 = 40$$

b. $\frac{1}{6}:1::x:1\frac{1}{2}$

$$1x = \frac{1}{6} \times \frac{3}{2}$$

$$1x = \frac{3}{12}$$

$$x = \frac{1}{4}$$

OR

$$\frac{\frac{1}{6}}{1} = \frac{x}{1\frac{1}{2}}$$

Proof:

$$\frac{1}{6}:1::\frac{1}{4}:1\frac{1}{2}$$

$$\frac{1}{6} \times 1\frac{1}{2} = 1 \times \frac{1}{4}$$

$$\frac{1}{\underset{2}{\cancel{6}}} \times \frac{\cancel{3}}{2} = \frac{1}{4}$$

$$\frac{1}{4} = \frac{1}{4}$$

$$\frac{\frac{1}{6}}{1} = \frac{x}{\frac{3}{2}}$$

$$1x = \frac{1}{6} \times \frac{3}{2} = \frac{3}{12} = \frac{1}{4}$$

c. $\dfrac{2.5}{x} :: \dfrac{5}{10}$ or $2.5:x::5:10$

$$5x = 25$$
$$x = 5$$

Proof:
$$2.5:5::5:10$$
$$2.5 \times 10 = 5 \times 5$$
$$25 = 25$$

d.
$$\frac{x}{3} = \frac{\frac{7}{9}}{\frac{21}{24}} \text{ or } x:\frac{3}{4}::\frac{7}{9}:\frac{21}{24}$$

$$\frac{21}{24}x = \frac{21}{36}$$

$$\frac{21}{24} \div \frac{21}{24}x = \frac{21}{36} \div \frac{21}{24}$$

$$\frac{\cancel{21}}{\cancel{24}} \times \frac{\cancel{24}}{\cancel{21}}x = \frac{\cancel{21}}{\cancel{36}}^{\,9} \times \frac{\cancel{24}}{\cancel{21}}^{\,6}_{\,1}$$

$$x = \frac{6}{9} = \frac{2}{3}$$

Proof:
$$\frac{2}{3}:\frac{3}{4}::\frac{7}{9}:\frac{21}{24}$$

$$\frac{2}{3} \times \frac{21}{24} = \frac{3}{4} \times \frac{7}{9}$$

$$\frac{42}{72} = \frac{21}{36}$$

$$\frac{7}{12} = \frac{7}{12}$$

e. $x:16::4:8$
$$8x = 64$$
$$x = 8$$

Proof:
$$8:16::4:8$$
$$8 \times 8 = 16 \times 4$$
$$64 = 64$$

f. $27:x::9:3$
$$9x = 81$$
$$x = \frac{81}{9}$$
$$x = 9$$

Proof:
$$27:9::9:3$$
$$27 \times 3 = 9 \times 9$$
$$81 = 81$$

g. $\dfrac{4}{5} :: \dfrac{20}{x}$
$$4x = 100$$
$$x = 25$$

Proof:
$$\frac{4}{5} :: \frac{20}{25} \text{ Cross multiply}$$
$$4 \times 25 = 5 \times 20$$
$$100 = 100$$

h. $\dfrac{7}{8} :: \dfrac{x}{64}$

$8x = 448$

$x = 56$

Proof:

$\dfrac{7}{8} :: \dfrac{56}{64}$

$7 \times 64 = 8 \times 56$

$448 = 448$

12. *Write the following Arabic numerals as Roman numerals.*

a. 8   VIII

b. 3   III

c. 21   XXI

d. 50   L

e. 5   V

f. 14   XIV

g. 101   CI

h. 1988   MCMLXXXVIII

Review

I = 1

V = 5

X = 10

L = 50

C = 100

D = 500

M = 1000

13. *Write the following Roman numerals as Arabic numerals.*

a. CIV   104

b. XL   40

c. MCMLXXXI   1981

d. XV   15

e. IV   4

f. XI   11

g. XXXIV   34

h. VII   7

14. *Change the following units to the indicated equivalents.*

Percentage	Decimal	Fraction	Ratio
a. **10%**	0.10	$\dfrac{1}{10}$	1:10
b. 65%	**0.65**	$\dfrac{13}{20}$	13:20
c. 25%	0.25	$\dfrac{1}{4}$	1:4
d. 0.2%	0.002	$\dfrac{1}{500}$	**1:500**

a. To change a percentage value to a decimal value, move the decimal point two places to the left and drop the percent sign:

$$10\% = 0.10$$

0.1 is read one tenth, or the fraction $\frac{1}{10}$. The ratio is formed from the fraction $\frac{1}{10}$.

b. The percent is determined from the decimal by moving the decimal point two places to the right and adding a percent sign. The fraction is determined by placing the decimal over 100, $\frac{65}{100}$, and, if possible, reducing the fraction, $\frac{65}{100} = \frac{13}{20}$.

c. The decimal is determined from the fraction by dividing the numerator by the denominator.

$$\frac{1}{4} = 4\overline{)1.00} \quad \begin{array}{r} .25 \\ \hline 8 \\ \hline 20 \end{array}$$

d. The fraction is determined from the ratio by writing the ratio as a fraction, namely 1:500 becomes $\frac{1}{500}$.

15. *Round the following numbers as indicated.*

Number	Round to the Nearest Whole Number	Round to the Nearest Tenth
a. 3.471	3	3.5
b. 8.94	9	8.9
c. 0.93	1	0.9
d. 0.082	0	0.1
e. 25.69	26	25.7

Number	Round to the Nearest Hundredth	Round to the Nearest Thousandth
f. 21.6107	21.61	21.611
g. 4.2187	4.22	4.219
h. 0.6709	0.67	0.671
i. 8.4653	8.47	8.465
j. 10.0294	10.03	10.029

Rounding Numbers:
The answer to dosage problems is not always an even number. In this textbook, any fractional number that is 5 or above is rounded up, and any number below 5 is dropped. Numbers may be rounded to the nearest whole number, tenth, or hundredth place. When measuring a liquid medication a hundredth is the smallest amount that can be measured in a syringe.

As you work through the dosage problems leave numbers to the thousandth place. Then round the final answer. This will result in greater accuracy.

As a review, look at the following number designations:

thousands, hundreds, tens, units · tenths, hundredths, thousandths
    4   6   5   3 · 8   9   4

The fractional numbers are the numbers that may be rounded. Apply the following guidelines to round the number correctly:

1. Mentally identify the place to which you are to round the decimal number.
2. Carry the decimal fraction one place beyond the number to which you are to round, and then round the identified number.
3. If the digit to the right of the identified number is less than five, drop that number and any number that might follow it.
4. If the number to the right of the identified number is five or more, increase the identified number by one and drop all the other numbers to the right of it.

For example, to round a number to the nearest tenth, carry the decimal fraction to the nearest hundredth place and round the number to the nearest tenth:

$$4.32 = 4.3 \qquad 6.49 = 6.5$$

To round a number to the nearest hundredth, carry the decimal fraction to the nearest thousandth place and round the number to the nearest hundredth:

$$2.321 = 2.32 \qquad 0.245 = 0.25$$

If you have mastered all of the problems in this self-evaluation test, you are ready to learn how to calculate dosage and solutions problems. If you fail to understand how to solve any group of problems, seek help from someone who understands the techniques, or refer to a basic arithmetic book. You *must* master the arithmetic, for it is basic to accurate dosage calculation.

1

The Metric System

OBJECTIVES

After completing this chapter, the student will be able to:

1. Name the basic units of the metric system used in nursing.
2. Interpret the abbreviations for metric units.
3. Write the units of weight and measure using the metric system abbreviations.
4. Convert larger metric units to smaller metric units.
5. Convert smaller metric units to larger metric units.

The metric system is a uniform system of weights and measures based on multiples of 10. Because of the ease of working within the decimal system, the metric system is used for most scientific and medical measurements.

The basic units of measure in the metric system are the *gram* (gm, g, or Gm), a unit of weight used for measuring solids; the *liter* (L or l), a unit of volume used for measuring liquids; and the *meter* (m or M), a unit of linear measure used to measure length or distance. Multiples of the basic units are designated by the prefixes deka- (10), hecto- (100), and kilo- (1000). Fractions of the units are designated by the prefixes deci- (0.1), centi- (0.01), milli- (0.001), and micro- (0.000001).

The four metric weights frequently used by nurses are stated from the largest to the smallest weight: the kilogram (kg); gram (g or gm); the milligram (mg or mgm); and the microgram (mcg or μg).

There are only two units of volume used by nurses. They are the liter (L) or the milliliter (ml). The cubic centimeter and the milliliter are considered equivalent and are used interchangeably: 1 ml = 1 cc.

The units of length used by nurses are the centimeter and the millimeter.

METRIC CONVERSIONS

Weight
Kilogram = kg or Kg
Gram = g, gm, or Gm
Milligram = mg or mgm
Microgram = mcg or μg

Liquid Volume
Liter = L or l
Cubic centimeter = cc
Milliliter = ml
Deciliter = dl

Length
Centimeter = cm
Millimeter = mm

SYSTEM	MULTIPLES OF THE UNIT			UNIT		DECIMAL POINT	FRACTIONS OF THE UNIT					
	THOUSANDS	HUNDREDS	TENS	UNIT		DECIMAL POINT	TENTHS	HUNDREDTHS	THOUSANDTHS	TEN THOUSANDTHS	HUNDRED THOUSANDTHS	MILLIONTHS
DECIMAL	0	0	0	0		.	0	0	0	0	0	0
METRIC	*KILO	HECTO	DEKA	*METERS, LITERS, OR GRAMS			DECI	*CENTI	*MILLI			*MICRO

* Measurements commonly used by health care providers.

EQUIVALENTS

Each of the following units differs from the next by 1000.

1000 g = 1 kg (100 g in each 0.1 kg)   1000 g = 1 kg
1000 mg = 1 g (100 mg in each 0.1 g)   0.001 g = 1 mg
1000 mcg = 1 mg (100 mcg in each 0.1 mg) 0.001 milligram or
                                                                    0.000001 g = 1 mcg

CONVERSION WITHIN THE METRIC SYSTEM

To change from a larger unit to a smaller unit:

kg to g
L to ml   *multiply by 1000*
g to mg
mg to mcg

This is the same as moving the decimal point 3 places to the right.

To change from a smaller unit to a larger unit:

g to kg
ml to L   *divide by 1000*
mg to g
mcg to mg

This is the same as moving the decimal point 3 places to the left.

Metric Weight

1 gram (g, gm, Gm) = 0.001 kilogram (kg or Kg)
               = 0.01 hectogram (hg or Hg)
               = 0.1 dekagram (dkg or Dg)
               = 10 decigrams (dg)
               = 100 centigrams (cg)
               = 1000 milligrams (mg)

Metric Volume

1 liter (L or l) = 0.001 kiloliter (kl or Kl)
               = 0.01 hectoliter (hl or Hl)
               = 0.1 dekaliter (dkl or Dl)
               = 10 deciliters (dl)*
               = 100 centiliters (cl)
               = 1000 milliliters (ml)

Metric Length

1 meter (m) = 0.001 kilometer
           = 0.01 hectometer
           = 0.1 dekameter
           = 10 decimeters
           = 100 centimeters
           = 1000 millimeters

---

* The deciliter (dl) is seen frequently in nutrition and laboratory value tables, e.g., mg/dl.

Symbols that may help you to remember:

larger ————————▷ smaller   to go from the larger measure to the smaller measure, move the decimal point the way the arrow points 3 places to the right.

smaller ◁———————— larger   to go from the smaller measure to the larger one, move the decimal point the way the arrow points 3 places to the left.

The wide end of the arrow represents the larger measure. The small end or point of the arrow represents the smaller measure and points in the direction the decimal point is to be moved.

Examples

1. *Convert liters to milliliters.*

$$4 \text{ L} = 4000 \text{ ml}$$

Multiply 4 by 1000 = 4000 ml   *OR*
Move the decimal point 3 places to the right: 4.000 L = 4000 ml

Liters are larger ————————▷ Milliliters are smaller

2. *Convert milliliters to liters.*

$$3000 \text{ ml} = 3 \text{ L}$$

Divide 3000 ml by 1000
$$\frac{3 \text{ L}}{1000)\overline{3000 \text{ ml}}} \quad OR$$
Move the decimal point 3 places to the left: 3000. ml = 3L

Milliliters are smaller ◁———————— Liters are larger

3. *Convert grams to milligrams.*

$$20 \text{ g} \times 1000 = 20{,}000 \text{ mg}$$

Move the decimal point 3 places to the right: 20.000 g = 20,000 mg

Grams are larger ————————▷ Milligrams are smaller

4. *Convert milligrams to grams.*

$$250 \text{ mg} = 0.25 \text{ g}$$

Divide 250 mg by 1000
$$\frac{.25 \text{ gm}}{1000)\overline{250.00 \text{ mg}}} \quad OR$$
Move the decimal point 3 places to the left: 250. mg = 0.25 g

◁————————

5. *Convert milligrams to micrograms.*

$$0.04 \text{ mg} \times 1000 = 40 \text{ mcg}$$

Move decimal point 3 places to the right $0.040 \text{ mg} = 40 \text{ mcg}$

6. *Convert micrograms to milligrams.*

$$25 \text{ mcg} \div 1000 = 0.025 \text{ mg}$$ $25. \text{ mcg} = 0.025 \text{ mg}$

Move the decimal point 3 places to the left

Note: Always place a zero in front of your decimal point when there is no whole number there. The zero gives emphasis to the decimal and helps prevent dosage errors.

PROBLEMS: METRIC SYSTEM CONVERSION

Cover the answers on the following page and convert the following units of measure.

1. *Liters to milliliters*

   a. 1 L   = _____

   b. 0.5 L   = _____

   c. 4.5 L   = _____

   d. 0.125 L   = _____

   e. 3.25 L   = _____

3. *Grams to milligrams*

   a. 2500 g   = _____

   b. 0.5 g   = _____

   c. 1.2 g   = _____

   d. 0.065 g   = _____

   e. 50 g   = _____

2. *Milliliters to liters*

   a. 500 ml   = _____

   b. 60 ml   = _____

   c. 5 ml   = _____

   d. 1300 ml   = _____

   e. 4225 ml   = _____

4. *Milligrams to grams*

   a. 1.5 mg   = _____

   b. 3 mg   = _____

   c. 0.5 mg   = _____

   d. 400 mg   = _____

   e. 6000 mg   = _____

5. *Kilograms to grams*

   a. 5 kg   = _____

   b. 30 kg   = _____

   c. 400 kg = _____

   d. 3.5 kg = _____

   e. 0.4 kg = _____

7. *Milligrams to micrograms*

   a. 0.6 mg   = _____

   b. 0.420 mg = _____

   c. 250 mg   = _____

   d. 125 mg   = _____

   e. 0.015 mg = _____

6. *Grams to kilograms*

   a. 50 g   = _____

   b. 25 g   = _____

   c. 2.2 g   = _____

   d. 2500 g = _____

   e. 425 g   = _____

8. *Micrograms to milligrams*

   a. 6 mcg   = _____

   b. 43 mcg   = _____

   c. 225 mcg   = _____

   d. 4513 mcg = _____

   e. 20,280 mcg = _____

ANSWERS: METRIC SYSTEM CONVERSION

1. *Liters to milliliters*

   a. 1 L   = 1000 ml

   b. 0.5 L   = 500 ml

   c. 4.5 L   = 4500 ml

   d. 0.125 L = 125 ml

   e. 3.25 L = 3250 ml

3. *Grams to milligrams*

   a. 2500 g   = 2,500,000 mg

   b. 0.5 g   = 500 mg

   c. 1.2 g   = 1200 mg

   d. 0.065 g = 65 gm

   e. 50 g   = 50,000 mg

2. *Milliliters to liters*

   a. 500 ml   = 0.5 L

   b. 60 ml   = 0.06 L

   c. 5 ml   = 0.005 L

   d. 1300 ml = 1.3 L

   e. 4225 ml = 4.225 L

4. *Milligrams to grams*

   a. 1.5 mg   = 0.0015 g

   b. 3 mg   = 0.003 g

   c. 0.5 mg   = 0.0005 g

   d. 400 mg   = 0.4 g

   e. 6000 mg = 6 g

5. *Kilograms to grams*

    a. 5 kg   = 5000 g

    b. 30 kg   = 30,000 g

    c. 400 kg   = 400,000 g

    d. 3.5 kg   = 3500 g

    e. 0.4 kg   = 400 g

7. *Milligrams to micrograms*

    a. 0.6 mg   = 600 mcg

    b. 0.420 mg   = 420 mcg

    c. 250 mg   = 250,000 mcg

    d. 125 mg   = 125,000 mcg

    e. 0.015 mg   = 15 mcg

6. *Grams to kilograms*

    a. 50 g   = 0.05 kg

    b. 25 g   = 0.025 kg

    c. 2.2 g   = 0.0022 kg

    d. 2500 g   = 2.5 kg

    e. 425 g   = 0.425 kg

8. *Micrograms to milligrams*

    a. 6 mcg   = 0.006 mg

    b. 43 mcg   = 0.043 mg

    c. 225 mcg   = 0.225 mg

    d. 4513 mcg   = 4.513 mg

    e. 20,280 mcg   = 20.28 mg

2

Reading Drug Bottle Labels

OBJECTIVES

After completing this chapter, the student will be able to:

1. Identify the trade or proprietary name of a drug.
2. Identify the generic name.
3. Identify the dosage strength of the medication.
4. Identify the number of tablets or volume of a drug in a bottle of medication.
5. Identify the usual dosage of the drug.
6. Identify special precautions listed that are relevant to law or safety.
7. Identify from drug labels that the drug is a controlled substance.
8. Identify the schedule for the controlled drug.
9. Identify reconstitution instructions for powdered or crystalline drugs.
10. Identify the route of administration for the drug.
11. Identify storage instructions.
12. Identify the manufacturer's name.
13. Identify the expiration date.

DRUGS

Drugs are manufactured under many different names. Nurses, physicians, and the general public may become confused by the fact that a variety of different names are used for one drug. Sometimes a brand name is so familiar and has been used for so long that nurses, physicians, and the public may think of the drug only by that name. Advertising practices make the brand names very familiar. The nurse needs to be familiar with the generic or nonproprietary name of each drug. This name never changes and may be used worldwide. It is written in lowercase letters. The proprietary or trade name is followed by a circled R, ''®,'' indicating that the name is protected by law and may only be used by the drug manufacturing company registering the name. Sometimes TM is used after the name indicating that this is the trademark of the manufacturing company.

Pictured on the following pages are some labels illustrating some of the many different proprietary names for the drug ampicillin for oral administration. Other pharmaceutical companies have still different names.

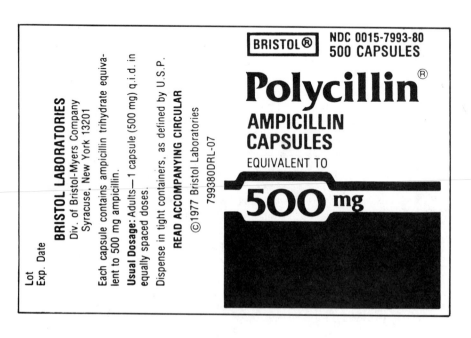

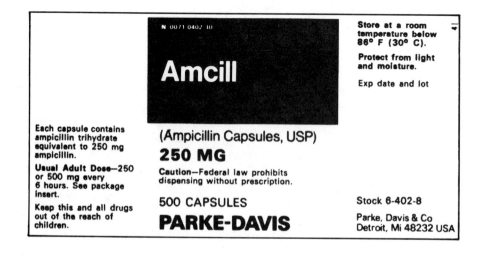

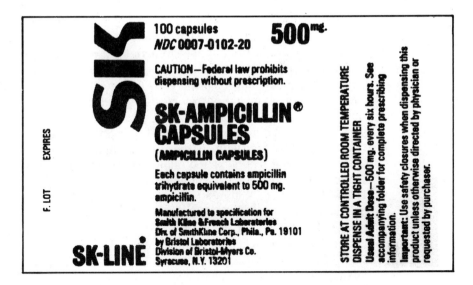

Bristol uses the name Polycillin ®
Parke-Davis uses Amcill ®
Smith Kline & French uses SK-Ampicillin ®*

Nurses must be certain they are using the correct drug. If you are in doubt about the drug, look it up in the Hospital Formulary, PDR, or nurse drug reference book. If you still cannot find the drug, call the pharmacist, who will be glad to assist you. Remember, it is better to ask questions than to make a drug error.

LABEL INFORMATION

The nurse must learn to read drug labels. The following will be found on the label:

1. Trade or brand name of the drug, frequently designated with ® at the upper right of the name, indicating that the name is registered and may be used only by the manufacturer who is the legal owner of the name.
2. Under the trade name will be the generic or official name. The drug may be ordered by either name, depending on the physician's preference or hospital regulation. Law requires that the generic name appear on the label.

---

* As of January, 1987, this line of ampicillin capsules has been discontinued.

3. On the label will be the strength of the capsule, tablet, or liquid, e.g., 25 mg capsules. This means each capsule contains 25 mg of drug. Drugs are usually manufactured in the strength most commonly ordered. Liquid drug labels will give the amount of drug in a given amount of solution, e.g., each 1 ml contains 300,000 U (*drug*) or each 2.5 ml dose contains 1 g of *drug* or 50 mg/ml, which means each 1 ml of liquid contains 50 mg of the drug.

4. The number of tablets or capsules that the bottle contains will be given. (Do not confuse this with the dose.) The total amount of liquid in an ampule or a vial will be stated, along with the total amount of drug in the vial or ampule, e.g., 60 ml or 100 capsules.

5. Usual dosage, e.g., 250 to 500 mg IV every 6 hours.

6. Special precautions may be listed: Do not give to children under 3 years of age; Federal law prohibits dispensing without a prescription; Controlled Substance Schedule Number, e.g., C_V *

7. If the drug is unstable as a liquid and is dispensed as a powder or crystals, mixing instructions are given.

8. The route of administration, for example, to be administered by intramuscular injection only.

9. Type of drug, e.g., capsule, tablet, spansule, suspension, etc.

10. Storage instructions are listed.

11. Manufacturer's name is given.

12. Expiration date is provided.

Use the information given in the following labels to complete the worksheet on page 35.

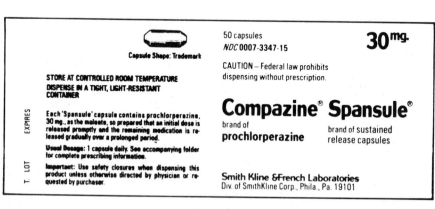

Bottle 1

* Controlled drugs: narcotics, sedatives, etc., fall into one of four classifications. These classifications are designated on the drug label by the symbols C_{II}, C_{III}, C_{IV} C_{IV} (See Tranxene label p. 33). This drug falls under the classification of C_V. The law designates different standards of control for drugs in each classification.

CAUTION—Federal
(U.S.A.) law prohibits
dispensing without
prescription.

See accompanying
literature for
dosage.

Keep Tightly Closed

Dispense in a tight
container.

NDC 0777-2315-05 Ⓡ

16 fl oz (1 pt) (473 ml)

M-148

ILOSONE®
LIQUID

**ERYTHROMYCIN ESTOLATE
ORAL SUSPENSION, USP**

125 mg per 5 ml

SHAKE WELL BEFORE USING

Refrigerate to maintain
optimum taste

Each 5 ml contains
Erythromycin
Estolate
equivalent to
125 mg
Erythromycin
in a pleasantly
flavored vehicle.

YC 4942 DPX
Manufactured by
DISTA PRODUCTS CO.
a Division of
Eli Lilly & Co., Inc.
Carolina, Puerto Rico 00630
a Subsidiary of
Eli Lilly & Co.
Indianapolis, IN, U.S.A.

Expiration Date/Control No.

Bottle 2

Each white
and gray capsule
bears the ⊇ and
the Abbo-Code CI
for identification.

See package
enclosure for
dosage and full
prescribing in-
formation.

_ Each capsule
contains:

clorazepate
— dipotassium
_ - - - - - - 3.75 mg

U.S. Pat. No.
_ Re. 28,315

100 Capsules

TRANXENE®

**3.75 Clorazepate
mg dipotassium**

Caution: Federal (U.S.A.)
law prohibits dispensing
without prescription.

Abbott
Pharmaceuticals, Inc.
North Chicago,
IL 60064, U.S.A.

New capsule size
adopted July, 1979.

Keep bottle tightly
closed. Dispense
in a USP tight
container.

Bottle 3

USUAL DOSAGE: See accompanying circular. Filled into container as a true solution, then cryodesiccated. To reconstitute, add 50 ml of 5% Dextrose Injection or Sodium Chloride Injection for slow intravenous injection. Discard unused solution after 24 hours.

6234806

50 mg | No. 3330

MSD

NDC 0006-3330-50

50 mg
INTRAVENOUS
SODIUM EDECRIN®
(ETHACRYNATE SODIUM, MSD)

50 mg Ethacrynic Acid Equivalent

CAUTION: Federal (U.S.A.) law prohibits dispensing without prescription.
SINGLE DOSE VIAL

MERCK SHARP & DOHME
DIVISION OF MERCK & CO. INC.
WEST POINT, PA. 19486, U.S.A.

Bottle 4

#228-1

RECOMMENDED STORAGE
STORE BELOW 86°F. (30°C.)
FOR INTRAMUSCULAR USE ONLY

NDC 0069-5460-74   9249

Vistaril®
hydroxyzine
hydrochloride

50 mg / ml
10 ml

INTRAMUSCULAR SOLUTION
CAUTION: Federal law prohibits dispensing without prescription.

READ ACCOMPANYING PROFESSIONAL INFORMATION

Each ml contains 50 mg of hydroxyzine hydrochloride, 0.9% benzyl alcohol and sodium hydroxide to adjust to optimum pH.

USUAL ADULT DOSE
Intramuscularly: 25—100 mg stat; repeat every 4 to 6 hours, as needed.

To avoid discoloration, protect from prolonged exposure to light.

U S Pat No. 2 899 436

P F I Z E R

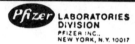 **LABORATORIES DIVISION**
PFIZER INC.,
NEW YORK, N.Y. 10017

P F I Z E R

10-1111-00-9
B-5344A

MADE IN U.S.A.

SIMKINS
7

Bottle 5

EXERCISES IN READING DRUG BOTTLE LABELS

Find each of the items listed on the sample drug bottle labels found on pages 32 to 34.

WORKSHEET: EXERCISE IN READING DRUG BOTTLE LABELS

	Bottle 1	Bottle 2	Bottle 3	Bottle 4	Bottle 5
1. Trade name					
2. Generic name or nonproprietary name					
3. Strength					
4. Total contents of bottle, i.e., number of capsules					
5. Usual dosage					
6. Special precautions					
7. Mixing instructions if applicable					
8. Route of administration					
9. Type of drug					
10. Special storage instructions					
11. Manufacturer's name					
12. Expiration date					

ANSWERS

ANSWER SHEET: EXERCISE IN READING DRUG BOTTLE LABELS

	Bottle 1	Bottle 2	Bottle 3	Bottle 4	Bottle 5
1. Trade name	Compazine Spansule	Ilosone Liquid	Tranxene	Sodium Edecrin	Vistaril
2. Generic name or nonproprietary name	prochlorperazine	erythromycin estolate oral suspension, USP	clorazepate dipotassium	ethacrynate sodium	hydroxyzine hydrochloride
3. Strength	30 mg capsules	125 mg/5 ml	3.75 mg	50 mg	50 mg/ml
4. Total contents of bottle, i.e., number of capsules	50 capsules	16 fl oz (1 pt) (473 ml)	100 capsules	50 mg of dry powdered drug. Single dose vial	10 ml
5. Usual dosage	1 capsule daily. See accompanying folder for complete prescribing information	See accompanying literature for dosage	See package enclosure for dosage and full prescribing information	See accompanying circular	Intramuscularly 25–100 mg stat; repeat every 4–6 hours, as needed
6. Special precautions	Federal law prohibits dispensing without prescription. Use safety closures when dispensing	Federal law prohibits dispensing without prescription	Federal (U.S.A.) law prohibits dispensing without prescription. Controlled substance schedule IV	Federal (U.S.A.) law prohibits dispensing without prescription	Caution: Federal law prohibits dispensing without prescription. To avoid discoloration, protect from prolonged exposure to light

	Drug 1	Drug 2	Drug 3	Drug 4	Drug 5
7. Mixing instructions if applicable	—	Shake well before using. (This drug is a suspension. The drug settles to the bottom)	—	To reconstitute, add 50 ml of 5% dextrose injection or sodium chloride injection for slow intravenous injection	—
8. Route of administration	Oral	Oral	Oral	Intravenous injection	Intramuscular solution
9. Type of drug	Sustained release capsule	Oral suspension	Capsule	Powder to be reconstituted	Liquid preparation for IM injection. Intramuscular solution
10. Special storage instructions	Store at controlled room temperature. Dispense in tight light-resistant container	Keep tightly closed. Dispense in a tight container	Keep bottle tightly closed. Dispense in a USP tight container	Discard unused solution after 24 hours	Store below 86°F (30°C)
11. Manufacturer's name	Smith Kline & French (SK&F) Laboratories	Dista Products Co., a Division of Eli Lilly & Co., Inc.	Abbott Pharmaceuticals, Inc.	Merck Sharp & Dohme	Pfizer Laboratories Division
12. Expiration date	NO EXPIRATION DATE IS GIVEN ON THESE LABELS BECAUSE THEY WERE "SAMPLE" LABELS. *REMEMBER TO CHECK THE EXPIRATION DATE!*				

3

Reading Syringe Calibrations

OBJECTIVES

After completing this chapter, the student will be able to:

1. Name the three syringes most frequently used in medication administration.
2. Read the calibrations on the three syringes.

SYRINGES

Syringes come in different sizes and are used for different purposes. The tuberculin syringe is a 1-cc syringe calibrated in minims and cubic centimeters (milliliters); very small amounts of solution may be measured with this syringe. Each line on the cubic centimeter scale stands for one hundredth of a cubic centimeter. The longer lines indicate tenths of a cubic centimeter. The minim scale is divided into 16 minims. This syringe is used for intradermal and subcutaneous injections. It may also be used to give an IM injection to small infants.

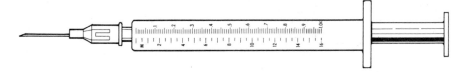

Tuberculin syringe calibrated in cubic centimeter and minim scales.

The insulin syringe is also a 1-cc syringe but is used only for administering insulin. The syringe is calibrated in units that must be matched to the strength of the insulin to be administered, i.e., a U100 syringe may only be used to administer U100 insulin (which has a strength of 100 units of insulin per cubic centimeter). Each line represents 2 units of insulin.

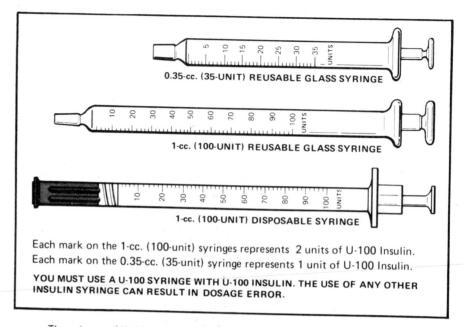

0.35-cc. (35-UNIT) REUSABLE GLASS SYRINGE

1-cc. (100-UNIT) REUSABLE GLASS SYRINGE

1-cc. (100-UNIT) DISPOSABLE SYRINGE

Each mark on the 1-cc. (100-unit) syringes represents 2 units of U-100 Insulin. Each mark on the 0.35-cc. (35-unit) syringe represents 1 unit of U-100 Insulin.

YOU MUST USE A U-100 SYRINGE WITH U-100 INSULIN. THE USE OF ANY OTHER INSULIN SYRINGE CAN RESULT IN DOSAGE ERROR.

Three types of U100 insulin syringes are pictured. The disposable and reusable 100 unit 1-cc syringes are used when giving larger doses of insulin. Each line represents 2 units of U100 insulin. The 35-unit 0.35 cc syringe is for administering small doses of insulin. Each line represents 1 unit of U100 insulin. (*From Directions for changing from U40 or U80 to U100 Iletin® [100 units of insulin per cc], published by Eli Lilly and Company, July 1973.*)

The 40 unit per cubic centimeter syringe should only be used with U40 insulin. Each mark on the 1-cc (40-unit) syringe represents 1 unit of U40 insulin.

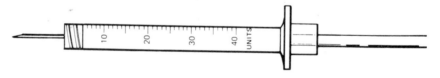

A 40-unit/cc syringe.

The standard 3-cc syringe is the syringe most frequently used. It is used for subcutaneous and intramuscular injections. The 3-cc syringe is calibrated in both minims and cubic centimeters. The minim scale is marked off in 1-minim increments up to 40 minims. The cubic centimeter scale is marked off in tenths of a cubic centimeter.

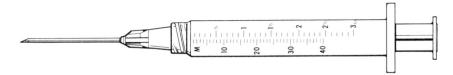

3-cc syringe calibrated in cubic centimeter and minim scales.

There are variations of the 3-cc syringe, such as the prefilled cartridge with an attached needle that inserts into a plastic case with a plunger for administration. These syringes are calibrated in tenths of a cubic centimeter, e.g., Tubex.

Larger syringes, from 5 to 50 cc, are available for larger quantities of medication or for irrigations. Look at each individual scale and determine the measurement represented by each line.

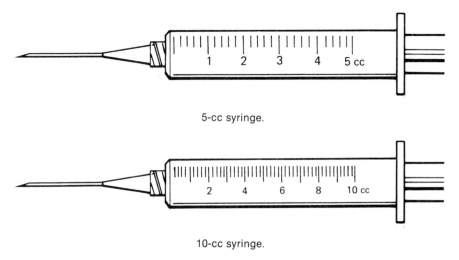

5-cc syringe.

10-cc syringe.

Syringes will be included with many problems throughout the text for you to shade to the correct dosage measurement.

4

Dosage Problems

OBJECTIVES

After completing this chapter, the student will be able to:

1. Compute dosage problems using either a formula or a ratio and proportion.
2. Identify the dosage strength of a drug from the drug label and use this information to set up and solve a dosage problem.
3. Define drug dose, drug strength, and vehicle.
4. Shade the medication cups and syringes to the correct dosage measurement.

Medications are prepared in either liquid, solid, or gaseous form. The pharmaceutical company places a specified concentration of the drug into a tablet, a caplette, or a liquid, along with binders, flavoring, and other substances. These ingredients are necessary to make the drug act in a specific manner within a certain time span. The form or *vehicle* in which the medication is prepared determines the route by which the drug can be administered, for example, orally, topically, by injection, or another route.

The physician prescribes the medication for the patient. The medication is supplied either as a unit-dose preparation or may be obtained from a stock supply of drugs. In either case it is necessary to check carefully for the correct drug, correct dosage, and for the proper route of administration. If the preparation is not packaged in the same dosage strength ordered by the physician, a dosage problem must be solved to determine the number of tablets or capsules or the amount of liquid that contains the dose prescribed.

General instructions for calculating the correct dosage of medication are:

1. Read the physician's order carefully.
2. Be certain you understand the order; if not, have the physician clarify the order for you. Never assume—be certain!

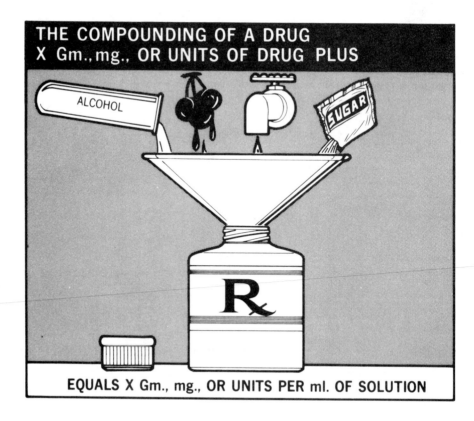

3. Next, compare the order with the drug and dosage on hand.
   a. Is this the correct drug?
   b. Is it the right form of the drug? Read the label carefully for form, i.e.,
      oral, intramuscular, or topical.
   c. Are the dosage units ordered and the dosage units available in the
      same unit of measure? (If the drug ordered and the drug available are
      not in the same unit of measurement you must convert the dosage
      ordered to the same unit of measurement as that of the available drug.)
4. Now set up your dosage problem and solve it.
5. Round answers to the nearest tenth.

   Either a formula or a proportion may be used to determine the amount
of medication containing the prescribed dosage. Choose the method that you
find easiest for you. *Do not try to use both methods but learn one method
thoroughly!*

METHOD 1: FORMULA

$$\frac{\text{Dose ordered (D)}}{\text{Drug strength on hand (H)}} \times \text{Vehicle (V)} = \text{Amount to give (G)}$$

$$\frac{D}{H} \times V = G$$

Dose ordered: Amount of drug ordered by the physician.

Drug strength on hand: Drug dosage from which to obtain the ordered dose.

Vehicle: Capsule, tablet, or liquid containing the dose on hand.

Amount to give: Amount of the vehicle to be given to the patient.

Example 1

The physician orders Keflex 750 mg.

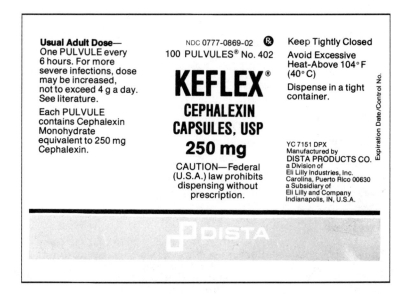

Step 1: Look at the medicine bottle label.

Each capsule of Keflex contains 250 mg.

Both the drug ordered and the drug on hand are in the same unit of measure: milligrams.

Step 2: Substitute into the formula.

$$\frac{D}{H} \times V = G$$

$$\frac{\text{Dose ordered}}{\text{Strength on hand}} : \frac{750 \text{ mg}}{250 \text{ mg}} \times 1 \text{ capsule} = G$$

$$\frac{\overset{3}{\cancel{750}}}{\underset{1}{\cancel{250}}} \times 1 \text{ capsule} = 3 \text{ capsules of Keflex}$$
$$250 \text{ mg each}$$

Be sure to label each number in the formula.
You may work the problem without canceling if you wish.

Step 3: Think: "I have 250 mg in one capsule; there are 750 mg in 3 capsules." Ask yourself if your answer is logical. Check your answer
by an alternate method of reasoning: 250 mg $\times$ 3 = 750 mg.

Step 4: Administer 3 capsules to the patient.

METHOD II: RATIO–PROPORTION

A ratio is a comparison between two related objects. When setting up a ratio
remember that you must compare like things to like things. Set up the first
ratio using information from the drug label. The second ratio is composed
of the drug ordered and the amount the patient is to receive (usually the
unknown).

Drug Label Information			**Dosage Desired**		
Strength on hand	:	Vehicle	:: Dosage ordered	:	Amount of vehicle to give
H	:	V	:: D	:	G

Example 2

The physician orders Keflex 0.75 g q6h (every 6 hours).

Step 1: Read the drug label (see label in Example 1). Each capsule contains Keflex 250 mg.

Step 2: The physician ordered 0.75 g Keflex. It is necessary to convert
grams to milligrams: 0.75 g $\times$ 1000 = 750 mg.

Step 3: Insert the label information into the ratio on the left and the
dosage desired into the ratio on the right. There is 250 mg in 1
capsule and you must give 750 mg. How many capsules will
you give?

$$\text{H} \quad : \quad \text{V} \quad :: \quad \text{D} \quad : \quad \text{G}$$
$$250 \text{ mg} : 1 \text{ capsule} :: 750 \text{ mg} : x \text{ capsules}$$

Multiply the means together and the extremes together. *Be sure to label all parts of the proportion.*

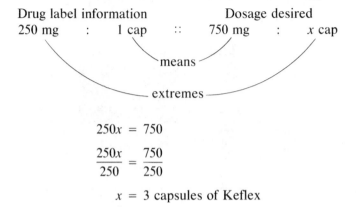

$$250x = 750$$

$$\frac{250x}{250} = \frac{750}{250}$$

$$x = 3 \text{ capsules of Keflex}$$

You may prefer to set up the proportions as fractions. The work is identical; to solve, cross multiply:

Drug label information   Dosage desired

$$\frac{H}{V} :: \frac{D}{G}$$

$$\frac{250 \text{ mg}}{1 \text{ cap}} \times \frac{750 \text{ mg}}{x \text{ cap}}$$

$$250x = 750 \text{ mg}$$

$$\frac{250x}{250} = \frac{750}{250}$$

$$x = 3 \text{ capsules}$$

Step 4: Check your answer by substituting it for x.

$$250 \text{ mg} : 1 \text{ cap} :: 750 \text{ mg} : 3 \text{ cap}$$
$$750 = 750$$

$$\frac{250 \text{ mg}}{1 \text{ cap}} \times \frac{750 \text{ mg}}{3 \text{ cap}}$$
$$750 = 750$$

Multiply the means and then multiply the extremes; if the two answers are equal, your answer is correct. *You can never be too cautious with medicine.*

Step 5: Administer three 250-mg capsules of Keflex to the patient.

Example 3

The physician orders Benadryl 50 mg.

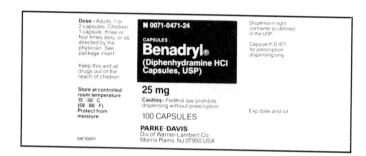

Set up your dosage problem by the method you prefer, using the four steps listed to prepare to administer the medication. After you have solved the problem, check your work.

$$\frac{D}{H} \times V = G$$

$$\frac{50 \text{ mg}}{25 \text{ mg}} \times 1 \text{ cap} = 2 \text{ capsules of Benadryl to be administered}$$

In this problem, the units are the same so you do not need to convert.

$$H \; : \; V \; :: \; D \; : \; G$$
$$25 \text{ mg} : 1 \text{ cap} :: 50 \text{ mg} : x \text{ cap}$$

$$25x = 50$$

$$x = 2 \text{ capsules of Benadryl}$$
to be administered

Remember the dosage you are to administer (capsules, tablets, milliliters, drams, teaspoons, ounces, etc.) is contained in the vehicle. You *do not* administer milligrams or grams. You administer *x* number of milligrams or grams or units of a drug in some type of vehicle (tablet, capsule, or liquid). This concept is illustrated in the figure below.

Smoke
Weed
everyday

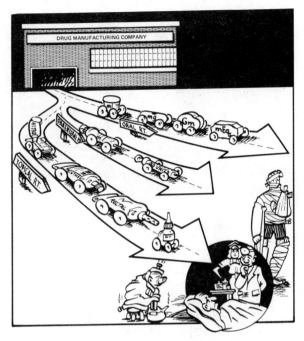

Vehicles for drug administration.

Example 4

The physician orders Depakene (valproic acid) 500 mg.

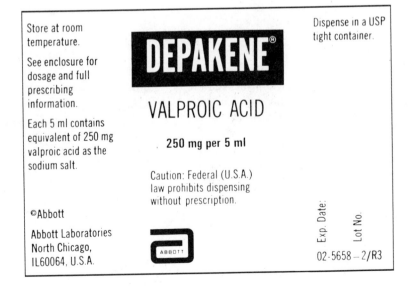

Store at room temperature.

See enclosure for dosage and full prescribing information.

Each 5 ml contains equivalent of 250 mg valproic acid as the sodium salt.

©Abbott

Abbott Laboratories
North Chicago,
IL60064, U.S.A.

DEPAKENE®

VALPROIC ACID

250 mg per 5 ml

Caution: Federal (U.S.A.) law prohibits dispensing without prescription.

ABBOTT

Dispense in a USP tight container.

Exp. Date:

Lot No.

02-5658 – 2/R3

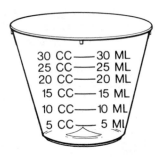

Fill medicine glass to the correct dosage.

Set up your dosage problem by the method you prefer. Work using the four steps outlined.

Formula method:

$$\frac{D}{H} \times V = \text{Dose to give}$$

$$\frac{\overset{2}{\cancel{500} \text{ mg}}}{\underset{1}{\cancel{250} \text{ mg}}} \times 5 \text{ ml} = 10 \text{ ml of Depakene to be administered}$$

Ratio method:

H : V :: D : G $\dfrac{250 \text{ mg}}{5 \text{ ml}} \diagup\!\!\!\!\diagdown \dfrac{500 \text{ mg}}{x \text{ ml}}$

250 mg : 5 ml :: 500 mg : *x* ml   *OR*

cross multiply

$$250x = 2500$$

$$x = \frac{2500}{250}$$

$$x = 10 \text{ ml of Depakene}$$

In this problem the vehicle is a liquid. The dosage strength is 250 mg per 5 ml of syrup. The patient is to receive 500 mg. The correct dosage for this patient is 10 ml of Depakene syrup. The medicine glass should be filled as indicated.

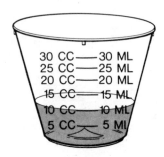

PROBLEMS: DOSAGE

Using the physician's order sheet and the drug labels for Problems 1 through 8, calculate the correct dosage to be administered. For problems involving liquid preparations, shade the medicine glass or syringe.

PHYSICIAN'S ORDER SHEET

PAGE NO. _____   PATIENT'S IDENTIFICATION

Date	Time	DOCTOR'S ORDER AND SIGNATURE		Orders Recorded	Completed or Discontinued		
					Date	Time	Init
		Doctor's Order and Signature					
		1 Vibramycin Capsules 0.2 gm po stat	1				
		2 Darvon Compound 65 1cap po q4h prn					
		3 Enduron 2.5 mg po qd	3				
		4 Dynapen 250 mg po q6h	4				
		Dr Dosage					
		Doctor's Order and Signature					
		5 Tobramycin sulfate 40 mg IM q4h	5				
		6 Cyanocobalamin 1,000 mcg IM today					
		7 cyclobenzaprine HCl 20 mg po TID X 7days					
		Doctor's Order and Signature					
		8 ampicillin Cap 500 mg po q6h	8				
		16	16				
		17 Dr Dosage	17				
		18	18				
		Doctor's Order and Signature					
		19	19				
		20	20				
		21	21				
		22	22				
		23	23				
		24	24				

DOCTOR: PRESS HARD YOU ARE MAKING 5 COPIES. TIME AND DATE YOUR ORDERS.
NURSING: PLEASE REMOVE COPIES OF DRUG ORDER FOR 60 MINUTE IMMEDIATE PICKUP.
T-1640 (Rev. 5/80)   ORIGINAL — DO NOT DETACH UNTIL FORM IS COMPLETED

1.

NDC 0069-0950-73

500 Capsules

Vibramycin®
Hyclate

doxycycline hyclate

equivalent to

100 mg†

doxycycline

CAUTION: Federal law prohibits
dispensing without prescription.

Pfizer LABORATORIES DIVISION
PFIZER INC., NEW YORK, N.Y. 10017

6505-00-009-5063

6286

RECOMMENDED STORAGE •
STORE BELOW 86°F (30°C)
Dispense in tight, light resistant
containers (USP).
†Each capsule contains doxycycline hyclate
equivalent to 100 mg of doxycycline.
MADE IN U.S.A. 3
doxycycline U.S. Pat. No. 3,200,149

READ ACCOMPANYING
PROFESSIONAL INFORMATION
USUAL DOSAGE — ADULTS: 200 mg on the first day
(100 mg every 12 hours) followed by a maintenance
dose of 100 mg a day.
IMPORTANT: This closure is not child-resistant.

2.

NDC 0002-0806-02
100 PULVULES® No. 369

Lilly C IV

Rx Pak

DARVON®
COMPOUND-65
PROPOXYPHENE
HYDROCHLORIDE
AND APC CAPSULES
USP

Caution—Federal (U.S.A.) law
prohibits dispensing without
prescription.

Usual Adult Dose—One PULVULE every 4 hours as
needed for pain.
See accompanying literature.
Each PULVULE Contains:

DARVON .... 65 mg.
  propoxyphene hydrochloride, Lilly
A.S.A. .... 227 mg. (3 1/2 grs.)
  aspirin, Lilly
Phenacetin .... 162 mg. (2 1/2 grs.)
Coffeine .... 32.4 mg. (1/2 gr.)
YB 5123 AMX
Mfd. by Eli Lilly & Co., Inc., Carolina, Puerto Rico 00630
a subsidiary of Eli Lilly & Co., Indianapolis, Ind., U.S.A.

100 Pulvules® DARVON® COMPOUND-65, Propoxyphene Hydro-
chloride and APC Capsules, USP
Keep Tightly Closed
Expiration Date/Control No.
Store at 59° to 86°F.
Lilly H06

FOR DISPLAY ONLY

100 Pulvules® DARVON® COMPOUND-65, Propoxyphene Hydro-
chloride and APC Capsules, USP
Keep Tightly Closed
Control No.
Store at 59° to 86°F.
Lilly H06

FOR DISPLAY ONLY

3.

| | | Dispense in a USP tight container. |

Each tablet contains:

Enduron (Methy-
clothiazide) ____ 5 mg

Usual adult dose: 2.5
to 10 mg once daily.

See package enclosure.

Each salmon-colored
tablet bears an ⊇
for identification as
an Abbott product.

Abbott
Pharmaceuticals, Inc.
North Chicago,
IL60064, U.S.A.

100 Tablets

ENDURON®

METHYCLOTHIAZIDE
TABLETS, USP

5 mg

Caution: Federal (U.S.A.)
law prohibits dispensing
without prescription.

Exp   Lot

©Abbott

03-0799—4/R8

4.

Lot
Exp. date of powder

STORE IN REFRIGERATOR: discard after 14 days

KEEP BOTTLE TIGHTLY CLOSED

SHAKE WELL BEFORE USING

Be sure to take each dose prescribed by your physician.

785664DRL-02

NDC 0015-7856-64

BRISTOL LABORATORIES
Div. of Bristol-Myers Company, Syracuse, New York 13201

Usual Dosage: Children weighing less than 40 Kg (88 lbs)—12.5 mg/Kg day in equally divided doses q 6h.
Adults and children weighing 40 Kg (88 lbs) or more—125 mg q 6h.

READ ACCOMPANYING CIRCULAR

To the Pharmacist: Prepare suspension at time of dispensing. 1. Shake container to loosen powder. 2. Measure 112 ml of water for reconstitution. 3. Add approximately one-half the water. Immediately shake vigorously. 4. Add remaining water and shake vigorously. Bottle then contains 200 ml of suspension. **Note:** This bottle is oversized to provide greater shake space for ease in reconstitution. Each 5 ml contains dicloxacillin sodium monohydrate equivalent to 62.5 mg dicloxacillin.

Normal handling may lead to lumps which are not dispersed with continued shaking.

BRISTOL® NDC 0015-7856-64
6505-01-024-8900

200 ml BOTTLE

Dynapen

LIFT HERE

**DICLOXACILLIN
SODIUM FOR ORAL
SUSPENSION**

EQUIVALENT TO

62.5 mg per 5 ml

DICLOXACILLIN

when reconstituted
according to directions.

NEW RED
COLOR
FORMULATION

CAUTION: Federal law prohibits
dispensing without prescription.

© 1977 Bristol Laboratories

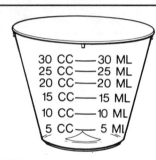

| 30 CC —— 30 ML |
| 25 CC —— 25 ML |
| 20 CC —— 20 ML |
| 15 CC —— 15 ML |
| 10 CC —— 10 ML |
| 5 CC —— 5 ML |

5.

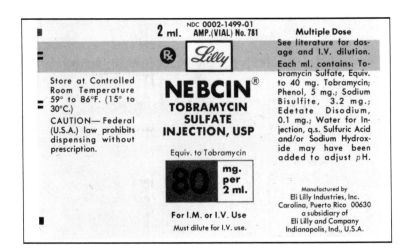

NDC 0002-1499-01
2 ml.   AMP.(VIAL) No. 781

℞ *Lilly*

NEBCIN®
TOBRAMYCIN SULFATE INJECTION, USP

Equiv. to Tobramycin

80 | mg. per 2 ml.

For I.M. or I.V. Use

Must dilute for I.V. use.

Store at Controlled Room Temperature 59° to 86°F. (15° to 30°C.)
CAUTION— Federal (U.S.A.) law prohibits dispensing without prescription.

Multiple Dose
See literature for dosage and I.V. dilution.
Each ml. contains: Tobramycin Sulfate, Equiv. to 40 mg. Tobramycin; Phenol, 5 mg.; Sodium Bisulfite, 3.2 mg.; Edetate Disodium, 0.1 mg.; Water for Injection, q.s. Sulfuric Acid and/or Sodium Hydroxide may have been added to adjust pH.

Manufactured by
Eli Lilly Industries, Inc.
Carolina, Puerto Rico 00630
a subsidiary of
Eli Lilly and Company
Indianapolis, Ind., U.S.A.

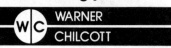

6.

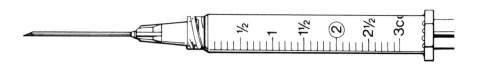

WARNER CHILCOTT LABS
Div of Warner-Lambert Co
Morris Plains, NJ 07950 USA

Each ml contains 1000 mcg cyanocobalamin. The solution also contains sodium chloride to make it isotonic and not more than 0.15% methylparaben and 0.02% propylparaben as preservatives. Sodium hydroxide or hydrochloric acid may have been added for adjustment of pH.

4119G011

N 0047-4119-10   **10** mL
Cyanocobalamin Injection, USP
(Crystalline Vitamin B₁₂)
1000 mcg per mL

W|C **WARNER CHILCOTT**

Caution—Federal law prohibits dispensing without prescription.
For intramuscular, subcutaneous or intravenous use.
Dosage—See package insert.
Store below 30°C (86°F). Protect from light.
Exp date and lot

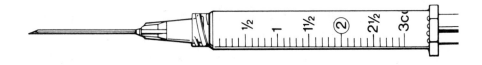

7.

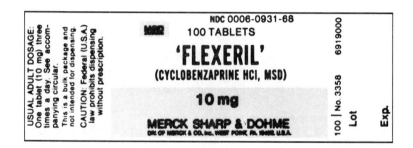

8.

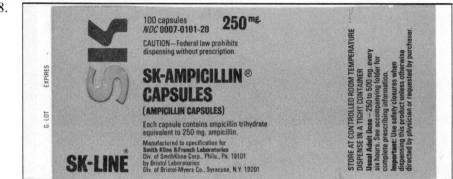

ANSWERS: DOSAGE PROBLEMS

1.

$$\frac{D}{H} \times V = G \qquad \text{Order: } 0.2 \text{ g} = 200 \text{ mg}$$

$$\frac{\overset{2}{\cancel{200} \text{ mg}}}{\underset{1}{\cancel{100} \text{ mg}}} \times 1 \text{ cap} = 2 \text{ capsules of Vibromycin}$$

2. Darvon Compound-65 is a compound of Darvon 65 mg, aspirin 227 mg, phenacetin 162 mg, and caffeine 32.4 mg. The order is for 1 capsule. Give 1 capsule; there is no problem to work. Just be sure you give the correct medicine. There are several different Darvon preparations.

3.
$$H \;:\; V \;::\; D \;:\; G$$
5 mg : 1 tablet :: 2.5 mg : x tablet

$$5x = 2.5$$

$$x = \frac{2.5}{5}$$

$$x = 0.5, \text{ or } \frac{1}{2} \text{ tablet of Enduron}$$

This tablet is grooved (scored), so that it may be cut in half.

4.
$$\frac{D}{H} \times V = G$$

$$\frac{\overset{4}{\cancel{250}} \text{ mg}}{\underset{1}{\cancel{62.5}} \text{ mg}} \times 5 \text{ ml} = 20 \text{ ml of Dynapen}$$

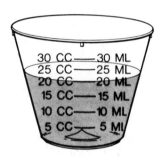

Dynapen is dicloxacillin. Observe that the instructions on the label say "Shake well before using." Be certain to read the label for special administration instructions.

5.
$$H \;:\; V \;::\; D \;:\; G$$
80 mg : 2 ml :: 40 mg : x ml

$$80x = 80$$

$$x = 1 \text{ ml of tobramycin}$$

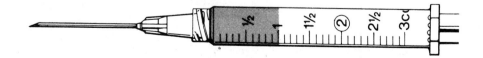

6.
$$\frac{D}{H} \times V = G$$

$$\frac{1000 \text{ mcg}}{1000 \text{ mcg}} \times 1 \text{ ml} = 1 \text{ ml of vitamin B}_{12}$$

Note that it was not really necessary to solve this problem because the desired dose and the "have" dose are the same.

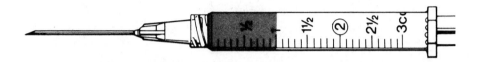

7.
$$\frac{H}{V} :: \frac{D}{G}$$

$$\frac{10 \text{ mg}}{1 \text{ tablet}} :: \frac{20 \text{ mg}}{x \text{ tablets}}$$

$$10x = 20$$

$$x = 2 \text{ tablets of cyclobenzaprine HCl}$$

Look carefully at the spelling of the name of the drug you are to give. Be certain you have the correct drug, as drug names are frequently very similar.

8.
$$\frac{D}{H} \times V = G$$

$$\frac{\overset{2}{\cancel{500} \text{ mg}}}{\underset{1}{\cancel{250} \text{ mg}}} \times 1 \text{ cap} = 2 \text{ capsules ampicillin}$$

5

Units and Milliequivalents

OBJECTIVES

After completing this chapter, the student will be able to:

1. Define unit.
2. Define milliequivalent.
3. Use a formula or proportion to solve dosage problems of drugs ordered in units.
4. Use a formula or proportion to solve dosage problems of drugs ordered in millequivalents.

Dosage problems involving drugs that are measured in units other than metric or apothecaries' system units are solved by the same formulas used for other dosage problems. The units or milliequivalents of a drug use tablets, capsules, or milliliters of liquid as the vehicle. These problems can be solved using the formula or proportion method that you have been using, with units or milliequivalents substituted into the dose ordered and strength on hand positions.

METHODS FOR SOLVING PROBLEMS INVOLVING UNITS AND MILLIEQUIVALENTS

A unit of drug is one that cannot be analyzed by chemical means. The drug is standardized by its effect on laboratory animals under controlled conditions. The strength is determined by the amount of drug required to bring about a desired effect in a laboratory animal. The strength of hormones and vitamins is measured in units. The abbreviation for unit is U.

Example 1

The physician orders penicillin G 600,000 units. The vial has been reconstituted to 500,000 U/ml. How much solution should be given? (Round the answer to the nearest tenth.)

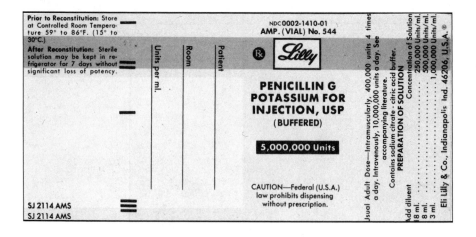

Method 1

$$\frac{D}{H} \times V = G$$

$$\frac{600{,}000 \text{ U}}{500{,}000 \text{ U}} \times 1 \text{ ml} = \frac{6}{5} = 1.2 \text{ ml of penicillin G}$$

Method 2

$$H \quad : \quad V \quad :: \quad D \quad : \quad G$$
$$500{,}000 \text{ U} : 1 \text{ ml} :: 600{,}000 \text{ U} : x \text{ ml}$$

$$500{,}000x = 600{,}000$$

$$x = 600{,}000 \div 500{,}000$$

$$x = 1.2 \text{ ml of penicillin G}$$

An equivalent is the unit of measure for chemical-combining activity of an electrolyte. The chemical-combining activity is based upon the number of available ionic charges (cations, anions) in solution. The concentration of electrolytes in biology is small and is, therefore, expressed as milliequivalents, $\frac{1}{1000}$ of an equivalent. One milliequivalent (mEq) of any ion can react completely with 1 mEq of any cation. Drugs used to maintain the body's electrolyte balance are usually measured in milliequivalents.

Example 2

The physician orders 80 mEq ammonium chloride to be added to 1000 ml D_5W. The strength on hand is 5 mEq per 1 ml. How much ammonium chloride must be added to the IV?

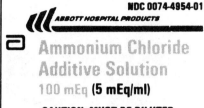

NDC 0074-4954-01

ABBOTT HOSPITAL PRODUCTS

Ammonium Chloride Additive Solution

100 mEq **(5 mEq/ml)**

CAUTION: MUST BE DILUTED FOR I.V. USE.

Warning: If crystals form, warm to room temperature to dissolve.

20 ml Partial-fill Single-dose Pintop Vial

Each ml contains ammonium chloride 267.5 mg and 2 mg disodium edetate (anhydrous) added as a stabilizer. pH adjusted with hydrochloric acid.
10.018 mOsm/ml (calc)   Approx. pH 5.0
Usual dose: See insert. Sterile, nonpyrogenic.
Use only if clear and seal is intact and undamaged.
Aseptically add to a suitable I.V. solution. Contains no bacteriostat; use promptly; discard unused portion.
Overfilled to compensate for product remaining after transfer of labeled amount.
Caution: Federal (USA) law prohibits dispensing without prescription.

Exp. Date
Lot No.

©Abbott   06-0954-3/R4-10/78   Printed in USA

Abbott Laboratories
North Chicago, IL60064, USA

Method 1

$$\frac{D}{H} \times V = G$$

$$\frac{\overset{16}{\cancel{80}} \text{ mEq}}{\underset{1}{\cancel{5}} \text{ mEq}} \times 1 \text{ ml} = 16 \text{ ml of ammonium chloride}$$

Method 2

$$H : V :: D : G$$

$$5 \text{ mEq} : 1 \text{ ml} :: 80 \text{ mEq} : x \text{ ml}$$

$$5x = 80$$

$$x = 16 \text{ ml of ammonium chloride}$$

PROBLEMS: UNITS AND MILLIEQUIVALENTS

Solve the problems below and shade each syringe to the correct dosage.

1. Give 5000 U of heparin. The label reads 10,000 U per ml.

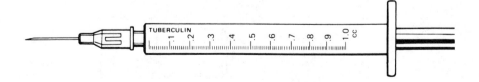

2. Give 7000 U of heparin. The label reads 10,000 U per ml.

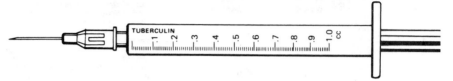

3. Give 500,000 U of Bicillin. The label reads 1,000,000 U per 5 ml.

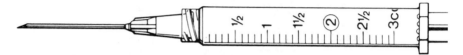

4. The doctor orders 150 U of a drug. If a vial contains 750 U per 5 ml, how much will you give?

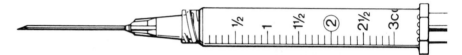

5. Give 50,000 U of sodium penicillin G from a multiple-dose vial containing 1,000,000 U per 10 ml.

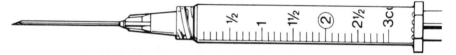

6. You are told to add 30 mEq of potassium chloride to an IV. The label on the potassium chloride vial reads 40 mEq per 10 ml. How many milliliters will you add?

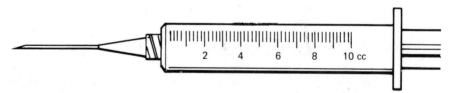

7. Add 20 U of Syntocinon to an IV. Syntocinon is supplied in 1-ml ampules containing 5 U per ml.

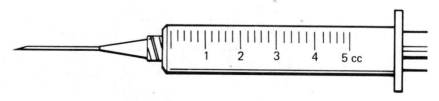

8. Give 15 mEq of potassium gluconate. Each tablet contains 5 mEq. How many tablets would you give?

ANSWERS: UNITS AND MILLIEQUIVALENTS

1. *Method 1*

$$\frac{5000 \text{ U}}{10,000 \text{ U}} \times 1 \text{ ml} = \frac{5000}{10,000} = 0.5 \text{ ml of heparin}$$

Method 2

$$10,000 \text{ U} : 1 \text{ ml} = 5000 \text{ U} : x \text{ ml}$$

$$10,000x = 5000$$

$$x = 5000 \div 10,000$$

$$x = 0.5 \text{ ml of heparin}$$

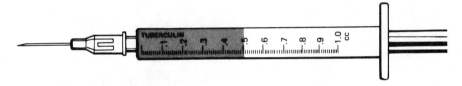

2. *Method 1*

$$\frac{7000 \text{ U}}{10,000 \text{ U}} \times 1 \text{ ml} = \frac{7000}{10,000} = 0.7 \text{ ml of heparin}$$

Method 2

$$10,000 \text{ U} : 1 \text{ ml} = 7000 : x \text{ ml}$$

$$10,000x = 7000$$

$$x = 7000 \div 10,000$$

$$x = 0.7 \text{ ml of heparin}$$

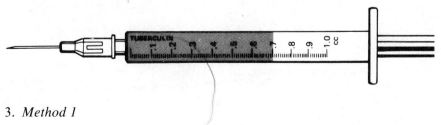

3. *Method 1*

$$\frac{500,000 \text{ U}}{1,000,000 \text{ U}} \times 5 \text{ ml} = \frac{2,500,000}{1,000,000} = 2.5 \text{ ml Bicillin}$$

Method 2

$$1{,}000{,}000 \text{ U}:5 \text{ ml} = 500{,}000\!:\!x \text{ ml}$$

$$1{,}000{,}000x = 2{,}500{,}000$$

$$x = 2{,}500{,}000 \div 1{,}000{,}000$$

$$x = 2.5 \text{ ml of Bicillin}$$

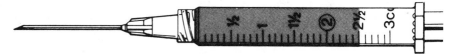

4. *Method 1*

$$\frac{150 \text{ U}}{750 \text{ U}} \times 5 \text{ ml} = \frac{750}{750} = 1 \text{ ml of the drug ordered}$$

Method 2

$$750 \text{ U}:5 \text{ ml}::150 \text{ U}:x \text{ ml}$$

$$750x = 750$$

$$x = 1 \text{ ml of the drug ordered}$$

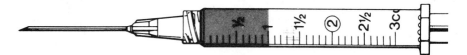

5. *Method 1*

$$\frac{50{,}000 \text{ U}}{1{,}000{,}000 \text{ U}} \times 10 \text{ ml} = \frac{500{,}000}{1{,}000{,}000} = 0.5 \text{ ml of penicillin G}$$

Method 2

$$1{,}000{,}000 \text{ U}:10 \text{ ml} = 50{,}000 \text{ U}:x \text{ ml}$$

$$1{,}000{,}000x = 500{,}000$$

$$x = 500{,}000 \div 1{,}000{,}000$$

$$x = 0.5 \text{ ml of penicillin G}$$

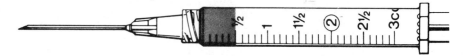

6. *Method 1*

$$\frac{30 \text{ mEq}}{40 \text{ mEq}} \times 10 \text{ ml} = \frac{300}{40} = 7.5 \text{ ml of potassium chloride}$$

Method 2

$$40 \text{ mEq}:10 \text{ ml}::30 \text{ mEq}:x \text{ ml}$$

$$40x = 300$$

$$x = 300 \div 40$$

$$x = 7.5 \text{ ml of potassium chloride}$$

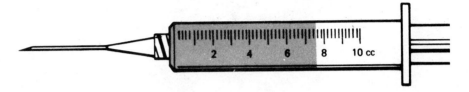

7. *Method 1*

$$\frac{20 \text{ U}}{5 \text{ U}} \times 1 \text{ ml} = \frac{20}{5} = 4 \text{ ml of Syntocinon}$$

Method 2

$$5 \text{ U}:1 \text{ ml}::20 \text{ U}:x \text{ ml}$$

$$5x = 20$$

$$x = 4 \text{ ml of Syntocinon}$$

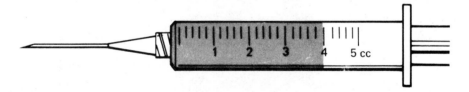

8. *Method 1*

$$\frac{15 \text{ mEq}}{5 \text{ mEq}} \times 1 \text{ tablet} = \frac{15}{5} = 3 \text{ tablets of potassium gluconate}$$

Method 2

$$5 \text{ mEq}:1 \text{ tablet}::15 \text{ mEq}:x \text{ tablets}$$

$$5x = 15$$

$$x = 15 \div 5$$

$$x = 3 \text{ tablets of potassium gluconate}$$

6

Insulin Administration

OBJECTIVES

After completing this chapter, the student will be able to:

1. Choose the correct insulin preparation.
2. Select the correct syringe for preparing the insulin dosage.
3. Shade the appropriate syringe to the correct dosage.
4. State the three things necessary for safe insulin preparation.
5. Calculate insulin dosage using a cubic centimeter syringe.

Insulin is a hormone necessary for carbohydrate metabolism in the body. It is produced in the pancreas. Insulin is prepared in so many units per milliliter. There is a trend to use only 100-unit insulin to cut down on dosage errors. However, insulin is still manufactured in other strengths: 20 U/ml, 40 U/ml, and 500 U/ml. The potency of the insulin does not alter the strength of the unit.

Be careful to choose the right kind of insulin. There are different insulin preparations; some are short-acting and must be given before each meal. Others have a medium-range action time and others are long-acting. Represented in the first figure are six varieties produced by Lilly, one manufacturer of insulin. Refer to a good pharmacology text for the action of the different types of insulin.

It is very important to measure insulin accurately to prevent serious problems. Insulin shock, coma, and death can occur from an untreated overdose of insulin. If insufficient insulin is received, the patient may develop hyperglycemia, leading to diabetic coma and death if left untreated. Insulin dosage can be calculated in milliliters or minims in the same manner as any other dosage problem, and may be given in a tuberculin or cubic centimeter syringe if absolutely necessary. (Many hospitals forbid this practice.)

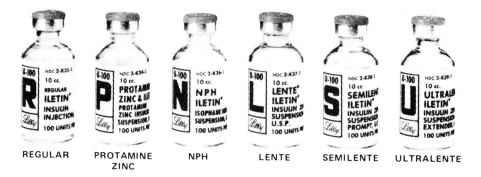

REGULAR   PROTAMINE   NPH   LENTE   SEMILENTE   ULTRALENTE
                ZINC

Insulin vials from Eli Lilly and Company. (From *Directions for changing from U-40 or U-80 to U-100 Iletin [100 units of insulin per cc], published by Eli Lilly and Company, July 1973.*)

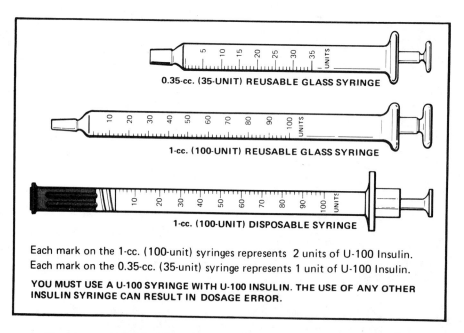

Each mark on the 1-cc. (100-unit) syringes represents 2 units of U-100 Insulin.
Each mark on the 0.35-cc. (35-unit) syringe represents 1 unit of U-100 Insulin.

YOU MUST USE A U-100 SYRINGE WITH U-100 INSULIN. THE USE OF ANY OTHER INSULIN SYRINGE CAN RESULT IN DOSAGE ERROR.

Three types of U100 insulin syringes are shown. The disposable and reusable 100 U 1-cc syringes are used when giving larger doses of insulin. Each line represents 2 U of U100 insulin. The 35-unit 0.35-cc syringe is for administering small doses of insulin. Each line represents 1 U of U100 insulin. (From *Directions for changing from U-40 or U-80 to U-100 Iletin [100 units of insulin per cc], published by Eli Lilly and Company, July 1973.*)

METHOD I: ADMINISTERING INSULIN USING AN INSULIN SYRINGE

The administration of insulin using an insulin syringe requires no calculations.

1. Read the physician's order and carefully match it with the correct type of insulin: for example, regular pork insulin, human NPH insulin. Eli Lilly and Company manufactures more than 25 different types of insulin (see illustration on pages 70 and 71). You must be able to choose the correct type and strength of insulin for your patient from the many types and strengths of insulin that are available. Note the U500 regular insulin (pork). Other manufacturers, such as Squibb and Nordish–U.S.A., each produce a line of insulins in U40 and U100 strength.
2. Obtain the correct insulin syringe. If the insulin to be given is U100 insulin, a 100 U/cc syringe is needed. Nearly all insulin prescribed contains 100 U of insulin per cubic centimeter. If another strength of insulin is prescribed, a specially marked syringe that matches the insulin strength must be used, for example, a U40 syringe with U40 insulin.
3. Draw the insulin into the syringe to the calibration of the insulin dosage ordered. Review syringes in Chapter 3.
4. Have a qualified person check the dosage and type of insulin prepared with the physician's order before you administer it.

Example 1

Question 1: The physician orders 20 U of Beef/Pork Semilente insulin at 7:30 AM and 5:30 PM. If the available Beef/Pork Semilente insulin is U100, what type of syringe would you use and how would you prepare it?

Answer: Use U100 Beef/Pork Semilente insulin and a 1-cc U100 syringe. Draw the insulin up to the 20 U calibration.

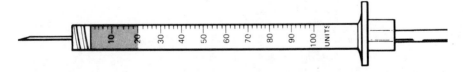

Twenty units of U100 insulin in a 1-cc disposable U100 syringe. (*From Directions for changing from U-40 or U-80 to U-100 Iletin [100 units of insulin per cc], published by Eli Lilly and Company, July 1973.*)

Question 2: If the available Beef/Pork Semilente insulin is U40, what type of syringe would you use and how would you prepare it?

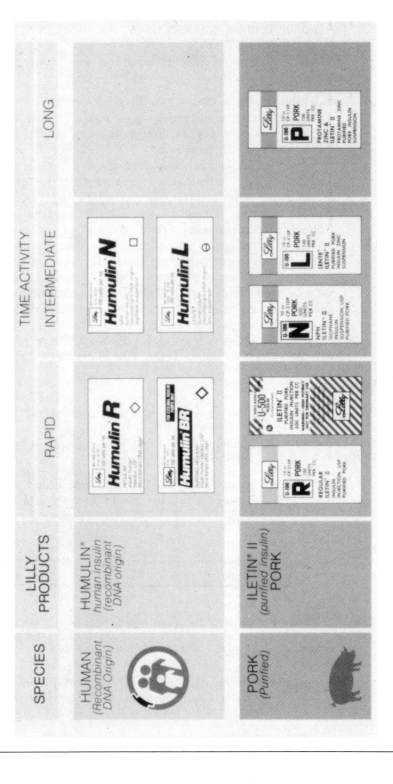

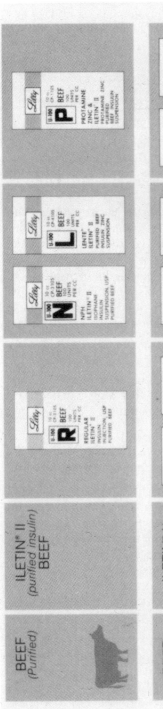
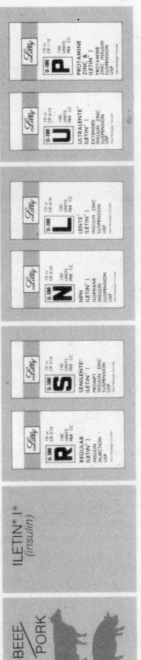

* Committed to diabetes care for over 60 years
* Supplier of the most extensive line of insulins
* First to introduce human insulin in the United States

WARNING

Any change of insulin should be made cautiously and only under medical supervision. Changes in refinement, purity, strength, brand (manufacturer), type (regular, NPH, Lente®, etc.), species source (beef, pork, beef-pork, or human), and/or method of manufacture (recombinant DNA versus animal-source insulin) may result in the need for a change in dosage.

*Iletin I formulations are also available in U-40 strength.

60-HI-2024-5   PRINTED IN USA   600715-89815   AUGUST 1986   © 1986, ELI LILLY AND COMPANY

Lilly insulins—the complete line. (Copyright 1986, Eli Lilly and Company.)

Answer: Use U40 Beef/Pork Semilente insulin and a 1-cc U40 syringe. Draw the insulin up to the 20 unit calibration.

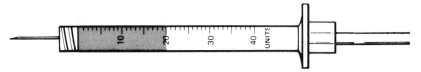

Twenty units of U40 insulin in a 1-cc disposable U40 syringe. (From *Directions for changing from U-40 or U-80 to U-100 Iletin* [100 units of insulin per cc], published by Eli Lilly and Company, July 1973.)

Compare the amount of insulin in each syringe. The strength of the U40 insulin is less than the U100 insulin, so more solution is required to give the same amount of insulin. The strength of the U100 insulin is greater, so less insulin is required to give the same amount of insulin. U40 insulin contains only two fifths as much insulin as U100 insulin per cc. This explains why it is so important to use the syringe with the correct calibrations.

Example 2

Sometimes two insulins must be given at the same time. This book does not cover the actual technique of adding air to a vial to withdraw a solution. This should be learned in a skills laboratory.

Question: Give 14 U of regular insulin and 26 U of NPH insulin at 7:30 AM. The hospital only stocks Humulin U100 insulin. What type syringe would you use and how would you prepare this dose?

Answer: Use U100 Humulin NPH insulin and U100 regular Humulin insulin and a 1-cc U100 insulin syringe. Draw 14 U of regular insulin into the syringe then draw 26 U of Humulin NPH insulin into the syringe. There is now a total of 40 units of insulin in the syringe.

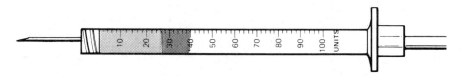

A U100 insulin syringe containing 26 units of Humulin NPH insulin (light shading) and 14 units of Humulin regular insulin (dark shading).

Follow hospital or agency policy about mixing insulin in one syringe. Some institutions do not allow 2 insulins to be mixed in one syringe.

METHOD 2: ADMINISTERING INSULIN USING A CUBIC CENTIMETER SYRINGE

Insulin may be given in a cubic centimeter syringe if necessary. Check the hospital or agency policy to see if this practice is acceptable. Because the tuberculin syringe is calibrated in hundredths, the insulin may be measured more accurately than with other syringes calibrated in cubic centimeters. Other cubic centimeter syringes may be used if no tuberculin syringe is available.

Insulin is prepared in a concentration of 100 U/cc solution or as a 40 U/cc solution. It also comes in solutions of 20 U and 500 U per cubic centimeter. These latter two strengths are rarely used.

Example 3

Question 1: The physician orders 20 U of Semilente Beef/Pork insulin. No insulin syringes are available. How could 20 U of Semilente Beef/Pork insulin be given in a tuberculin syringe? Set up a dosage problem using U100 insulin, calculate the dosage and shade the tuberculin syringe to the correct calibration.

Answer:

$$\frac{20\ U}{100\ U} \times 1\ cc = \frac{2}{10}$$

$$= 0.2\ cc$$

$$\frac{100\ U}{1\ cc} = \frac{20\ U}{x\ cc}$$

$$100x = 20$$

$$x = 0.2\ cc$$

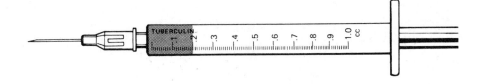

Question 2: Set up a dosage problem using U40 insulin. Administer 20 units of insulin.

Answer: 1
$$\frac{\cancel{20}\text{ U}}{\cancel{40}\text{ U}} \times 1 \text{ cc} = \frac{1}{2}$$
2
$$= 0.5 \text{ cc}$$

$$\frac{40 \text{ U}}{1 \text{ cc}} = \frac{20 \text{ U}}{x \text{ cc}}$$

$$40x = 20$$

$$x = 0.5 \text{ cc}$$

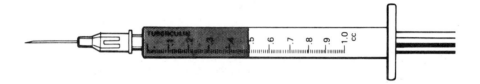

Compare the amount of insulin in each syringe. There is a smaller amount, 0.2 cc of U100 insulin, compared to 0.5 cc of U40 insulin, due to the difference in strength of the two insulins. Insulin used improperly can cause harm to the patient. Always use great care when administering insulin.

PROBLEMS: INSULIN ADMINISTRATION

Solve all problems using an insulin syringe and a tuberculin syringe. Shade insulin and tuberculin syringes to the correct dosage.

1. The physician orders 30 U of U40 Regular insulin stat.
   Type of syringe?
   Type of insulin?
   How would you prepare this dose in an insulin syringe? In a tuberculin syringe? Show dosage calculations.

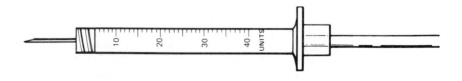

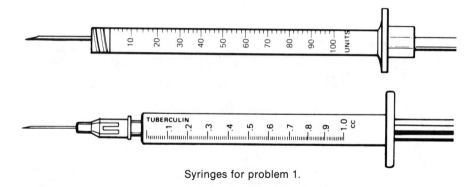

Syringes for problem 1.

2. The physician orders 90 U of U100 NPH insulin qd.
   Type of syringe?
   Type of insulin?
   How would you prepare this dose in an insulin syringe? In a tuberculin syringe?

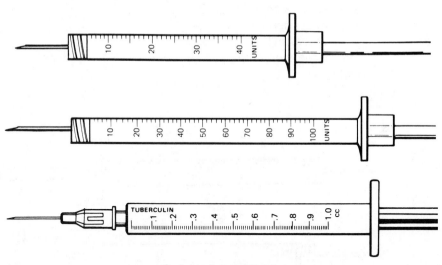

Syringes for problem 2.

3. The physician orders 46 U of NPH Humulin insulin to be administered before breakfast. It is available as U100/ml Humulin N insulin.
   Type of syringe?
   Type of insulin?
   How would you prepare this dose in an insulin syringe? In a tuberculin syringe?

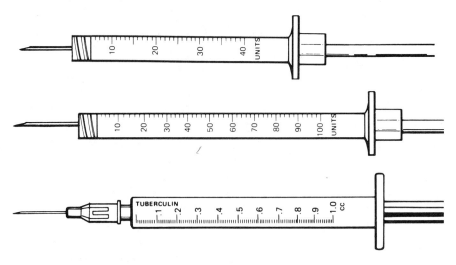

Syringes for problem 3.

4. The physician orders 15 U of Monotard insulin at 7:30 AM. It is available as U100/ml Monotard insulin.
   Type of syringe?
   Type of insulin?
   How would you prepare this dose in an insulin syringe? In a tuberculin syringe?

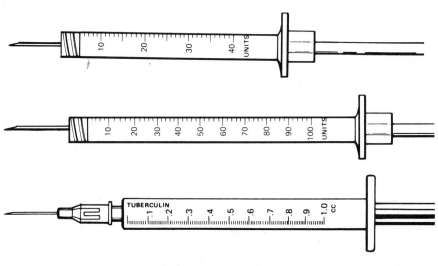

Syringes for problem 4.

5. The physician orders 56 U of Protamine Zinc Insulin qAM (every morn-
   ing). It is available as U100/ml Protamine Zinc Insulin.
   Type of syringe?
   Type of insulin?
   How would you prepare this insulin in an insulin syringe?
   In a tuberculin syringe?

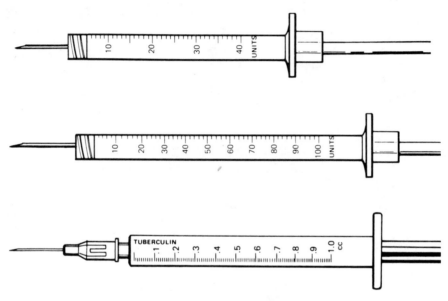

Syringes for problem 5.

ANSWERS: INSULIN ADMINISTRATION

1. Use a U40 insulin syringe.
   Use 40-U/ml Regular insulin.
   Draw 40-U/ml Regular insulin up to the 30 U mark on a U40 syringe.

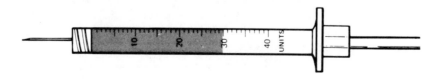

If you were using a tuberculin syringe you would determine the volume in milliliters as follows:

$$\frac{30 \text{ U}}{40 \text{ U}} \times 1 \text{ ml} = \frac{3}{4}$$

$$= 0.75 \text{ ml}$$

$$40 \text{ U}:1 \text{ ml}::30 \text{ U}:x \text{ ml}$$

$$40x = 30$$

$$x = 0.75 \text{ ml}$$

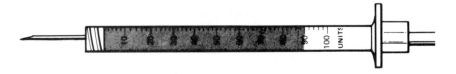

2. Use a U100 insulin syringe.
   Use 100-U/ml NPH insulin.
   Draw 100-U/ml NPH insulin up to the 90 U mark on a U100 syringe.

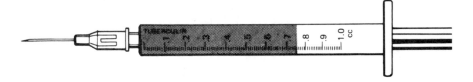

If you were using a tuberculin syringe, you would determine the volume in milliliters as follows:

$$\frac{90 \text{ U}}{100 \text{ U}} \times 1 \text{ ml} = \frac{9}{10}$$

$$= 0.9 \text{ ml}$$

$$100 \text{ U}:1 \text{ ml}::90 \text{ U}:x \text{ ml}$$

$$100x = 90$$

$$x = 0.9 \text{ ml}$$

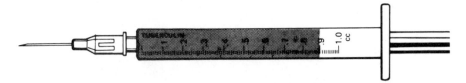

3. Use a U100 insulin syringe.
   Use 100-U/ml Humulin insulin.
   Draw 100-U/ml Humulin insulin up to the 46 U mark on a U100 syringe.

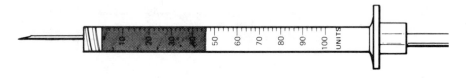

If you are using a tuberculin syringe, calculate milliliters as follows:

$$\frac{46 \text{ U}}{100 \text{ U}} \times 1 \text{ ml} = \frac{46}{100}$$

$$= 0.46 \text{ ml}$$

100 U:1 ml::46 U:x ml

$$100x = 46$$

$$x = 0.46$$

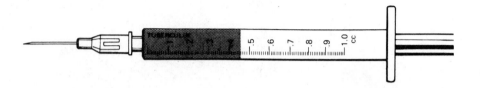

4. Use a U100 insulin syringe.
   Use 100-U/ml Monotard insulin.
   Draw 100-U/ml Monotard insulin up to the 15 U mark on a U100 syringe.

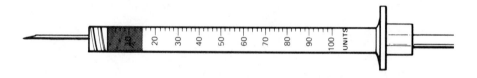

If you are using a tuberculin syringe, calculate milliliters as follows:

$$\frac{15 \text{ U}}{100 \text{ U}} \times 1 \text{ ml} = \frac{15}{100}$$

$$= 0.15 \text{ ml}$$

100 U:1 ml::15 U:x ml

$$100x = 15$$

$$x = 0.15 \text{ ml}$$

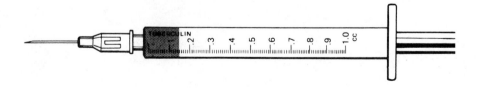

5. Use a U100 insulin syringe.
   Use 100-U/ml Protamine Zinc Insulin (PZI).

Draw 100-U/ml PZI insulin up to the 56 U mark on a U100 syringe.

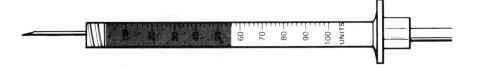

If you are using a tuberculin syringe, calculate milliliters as follows:

$$\frac{56 \text{ U}}{100 \text{ U}} \times 1 \text{ ml} = \frac{56}{100}$$

$$= 0.56 \text{ ml}$$

$$100 \text{ U}:1 \text{ ml}::56 \text{ U}:x \text{ ml}$$

$$100x = 56$$

$$x = 0.56 \text{ ml}$$

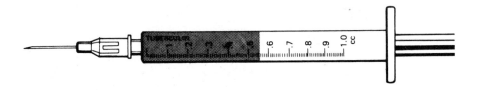

7

Reconstituting Drugs in Powdered or Crystalline Form

OBJECTIVES

After completing this chapter, the student will be able to:

1. Select the correct diluent.
2. State the correct amount of diluent needed to reconstitute the drug.
3. Follow the mixing instructions stated on the bottle to prepare the solution.
4. Find the dosage strength of the solution on the label and use it to complete the dosage problem.
5. Define drug displacement.
6. Identify storage instructions.
7. Identify the stability period of the drug.
8. Choose the correct strength to mix a drug when several choices of mixing instructions are given.

METHODS

Some drugs are unstable in liquid form. These drugs are dispensed in crystalline or powdered form. The nurse must add the diluent according to the manufacturer's instructions. After carefully following the mixing instructions, the nurse must then look for the strength of the reconstituted drug and administer the correct dosage. The usual diluents are normal saline or sterile water for injection. The drugs are dispensed in either single dose or multidose vials.

Look at the label. Easy to follow directions are included to prepare the solution. Simply follow the directions step by step.

1. Look at the Keflin label.

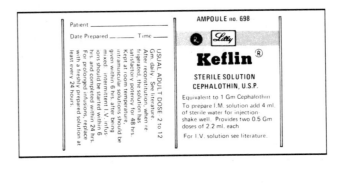

Note: This label is not currently in use. Keflin is usually given IV. Used by special permission of Eli Lilly and Company.

2. Mix the drug as instructed: add 4 ml of sterile water for injection, and SHAKE WELL. Your solution is now made. You do not need to do anything more with these instructions.
3. Now look for the dosage strength of the solution of Keflin. You will see that the solution you just mixed provides two 0.5-g doses of 2.2 ml each. Use these figures to compute your dosage.

If the doctor has ordered 0.5 g, you must give 2.2 ml.
If the doctor has ordered 0.25 g, you must give 1.1 ml.

$$\frac{\overset{1}{\cancel{0.25}} g}{\underset{2}{\cancel{0.5}} g} \times 2.2 \text{ ml} = 1.1 \text{ ml}$$

If the doctor has ordered 1 g, you must give 4.4 ml.

$$\frac{\overset{2}{\cancel{1} g}}{\underset{1}{\cancel{0.5} g}} \times 2.2 \text{ ml} = 4.4 \text{ ml}$$

DISPLACEMENT

When 1 g of Keflin is mixed with 4 ml of sterile water for injection, the resulting solution contains two 0.5-g doses of 2.2 ml each, so that the total solution measures 4.4 ml. The extra 0.4 ml volume results from the space required by the 1 g of Keflin. The pharmaceutical company allows for the drug displacement by adding the extra 0.4 ml of solution to the dosage strength of the drug, 1 g of Keflin per 4.4 ml. The amount of drug displacement is different for each drug.

DISPLACEMENT

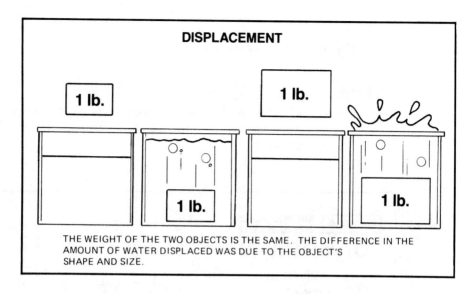

THE WEIGHT OF THE TWO OBJECTS IS THE SAME. THE DIFFERENCE IN THE AMOUNT OF WATER DISPLACED WAS DUE TO THE OBJECT'S SHAPE AND SIZE.

In some instances, the hospital may not stock the dosage strength you need, but will send a unit dose vial containing a larger dose than you will give. The pharmaceutical company assumes that you are going to give the entire contents of the vial, but you may only need a portion of the vial. After mixing the drug, measure the resulting solution and *calculate the dosage from the measured amount*, remembering there is drug displacement in all solutions. The larger the quantity of drug, the greater the displacement.

Example 1

Loridine 1 g
Add 2.5 ml of sterile water.
The finished solution measures 3.3 ml.
How much displacement occurred?

$$\begin{array}{r} 3.3 \text{ ml total solution} \\ -\ \underline{2.5} \text{ ml solution added} \\ 0.8 \text{ ml displacement} \end{array}$$

To give 0.5 g of Loridine, how much solution will you give?

$$\frac{0.5 \text{ g}}{1} \times 3.3 \text{ ml} = \frac{1.65}{1}$$
$$= 1.65 \text{ ml}$$

$$1 \text{ g} : 3.3 \text{ ml} :: 0.5 \text{ g} : x \text{ ml}$$
$$1\,x = 1.65 \text{ ml}$$

Remember, if the pharmaceutical company does not list the amount of solution in the bottle, and you are not going to give all of the solution:

1. Measure the contents of the bottle.

2. Using this measurement, calculate the amount of solution containing the correct dosage (amount ordered).

Example 2

Questions: Using the information given on the Polycillin-N (ampicillin) label, answer the following questions and solve the dosage problems.

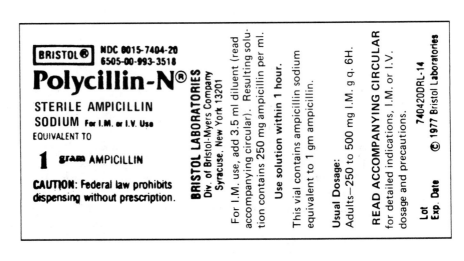

a. How much diluent must you add?
b. What is the dosage strength of this solution?
c. If the physician orders 250 mg, how much solution will you give?
d. If the physician orders 500 mg, how much solution will you give?
e. If the physician orders 1 g, how much solution will you give?

Answers: a. The amount of diluent to add is 3.5 ml.
b. The dosage strength is 250 mg/ml.
c. To give 250 mg, you would give 1 ml.
d. To give 500 mg, you would give 2 ml.

$$\frac{\overset{2}{\cancel{500}}\ mg}{\underset{1}{\cancel{250}}\ mg} \times 1\ ml = 2\ ml$$

$$250\ mg : 1\ ml :: 500\ mg : x\ ml$$
$$250x = 500$$
$$x = 2\ ml$$

e. To give 1 g, you would give 4 ml.
First convert: 1 g = 1000 mg

$$\frac{\overset{4}{\cancel{1000}\text{ mg}}}{\underset{1}{\cancel{250}\text{ mg}}} \times 1\text{ ml} = 4\text{ ml}$$

$$250\text{ mg}:1\text{ ml}::1000\text{ mg}:x\text{ ml}$$
$$250x = 1000$$
$$x = 4\text{ ml}$$

Example 3

The instructions for mixing penicillin G potassium for injection 5,000,000 U is different. You have a choice of three different strengths for mixing this drug. Choose the dilution that will give a concentration close to the amount of drug to be given. If the physician orders 250,000 U for the patient, mix the penicillin G by adding 18 ml of diluent. The resulting solution will then contain a dosage strength of 250,000 U/ml of solution. If the physician orders 1,000,000 U of penicillin G, you would add only 3 ml of diluent. The resulting dosage strength will be 1,000,000 U/ml.

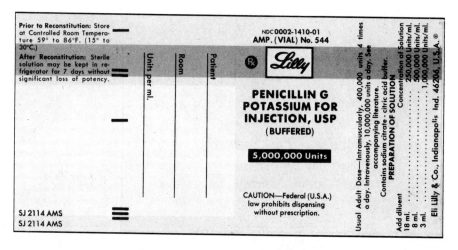

Questions: a. How much diluent must you add to the vial (ampule) if the doctor orders 500,000 U?
  b. How much solution will you give to administer 500,000 U?

If the physician orders 750,000 U to be given IM
  c. How much diluent would you add?
  d. How much solution will you administer to the patient?

One and a half milliliters of solution is within acceptable standards for an IM injection. The solution is not so concentrated that the injection would be irritating to the intramuscular tissue, or so dilute that the volume of the solution would be too large. The nurse must choose the dilution nearest to the dose ordered. Had the nurse chosen to dilute the penicillin with 3 ml of diluent, the dose of penicillin would have been 0.75 ml, an acceptable amount. Had the nurse chosen to dilute the penicillin with 18 ml of the diluent, the dose to give would have been 3 ml, a larger than necessary amount that would be more painful to the patient.

Answers: a. The amount of diluent to add is 8 ml.
b. You will give 1 ml. The dosage strength is 500,000 U/ml.
c. Use 8 ml diluent to make a solution of 500,000 U/ml.
d. You will administer 1.5 ml:

$$\frac{\overset{3}{\cancel{750,000}} \text{ U}}{\underset{2}{\cancel{500,000}} \text{ U}} \times 1 \text{ ml} = \frac{3}{2} = 1.5 \text{ ml of penicillin}$$

OR

$$500,000 \text{ U}:1 \text{ ml}::750,000 \text{ U}:x \text{ ml}$$
$$500,000 \ x = 750,000$$
$$x = \frac{750,000}{500,000} = \frac{3}{2} = 1.5 \text{ ml}$$

PROBLEMS: MIXING POWDERED DRUGS

1. The physician orders sodium oxacillin 250 mg IM.

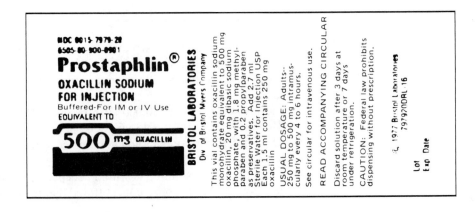

a. How much diluent must you add?

b. What diluent will you use?

c. After mixing, how many days is the solution stable?

d. How much solution will you give? Indicate this amount by shading the syringe below.

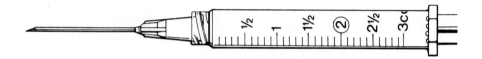

2. The physician orders Prostaphlin 500 mg (see label for problem 1).

a. How much solution will you give? Indicate this amount on the syringe below.

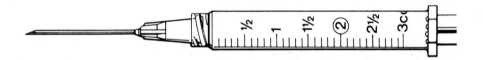

3. Referring to the label, prepare Ancef 1 g for IM injection.

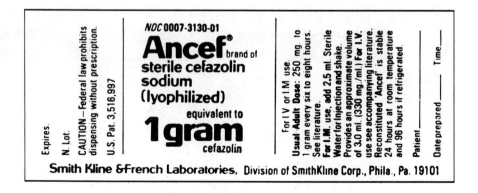

a. How much diluent will you use?

b. What diluent will you use?

c. How long is this reconstituted solution stable?

d. Administer 660 mg. How much solution will you give? Indicate this amount on the syringe below.

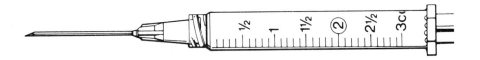

e. To administer 1 g, how much solution will you give? Indicate this amount on the syringe below.

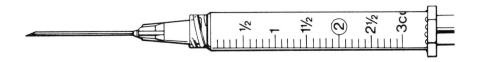

4. Referring to the label, prepare 1 g cefazolin sodium for IV administration.

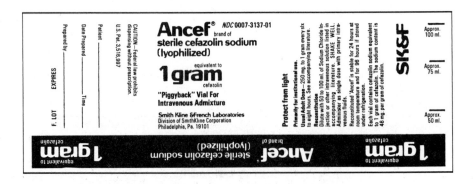

a. How much diluent must you add?

b. What diluent can be used?

c. How long is this solution stable?

5. Referring to the label, prepare 1 g Cefadyl for IV administration.

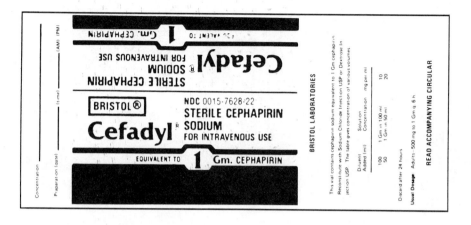

   a. How much diluent must you add?

   b. What diluent can you use?

   c. What special instructions are given?

   d. What is the usual dosage?

   e. What is the dosage strength of each of the solutions you may prepare?

6. Referring to the label, administer 0.5 g of ampicillin-N IM stat (at once) and q6h (every 6 hours).

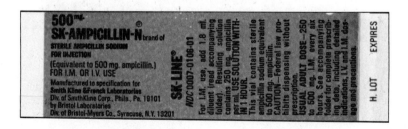

   a. How much diluent will you add?

   b. What is the usual adult dose?

   c. How much solution will you administer per dose?

7. Referring to the label, administer Polymox 0.25 g po q8h (by mouth every 8 hours). You have a unit dose bottle of Polymox.

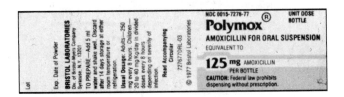

   a. How much diluent will you add?

   b. What diluent will you use?

   c. How long is the reconstituted solution stable?

   d. How many milliliters are necessary to give 0.25 g of Polymox?

8. Referring to the label, administer Kefzol 750 mg IM q6h.

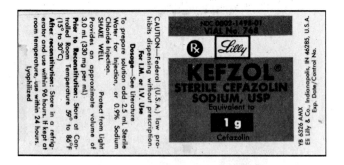

   a. How would you prepare this solution?

   b. What is the dosage strength after reconstitution?

   c. What are the storage instructions?

   d. How many milliliters of Kefzol are necessary to administer 750 mg?

9. Physician's order: Administer 200,000 U of penicillin G potassium IM q6h. You have a 1 million-unit bottle of Pfizerpen. (See label for instructions.)

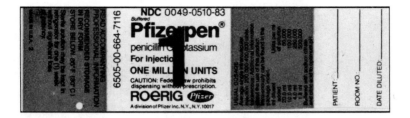

a. How much diluent will you add to make the desired strength?

b. What is the dosage strength of the solution you mixed?

c. How much Pfizerpen will you need to administer 200,000 U per dose?

10. Physician's order: Administer 350,000 U of penicillin G potassium IM q6h. (See label from question 9.)

a. What is the dosage strength of the solution you mixed?

b. How much diluent did you use?

c. How much Pfizerpen will you need to administer 350,000 U per dose?

ANSWERS: MIXING POWDERED DRUGS

1. a. 2.7 ml

   b. Sterile water for injection U.S.P.

   c. Discard solution after 3 days at room temperature or 7 days under refrigeration

   d. 1.5 ml of sodium oxacillin

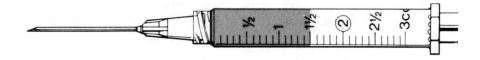

2. a. 3 ml

$$\frac{\overset{2}{\cancel{500}\text{ mg}}}{\underset{1}{\cancel{250}\text{ mg}}} \times 1.5\text{ ml} = 3.0\text{ ml}$$
of Prostaphlin

250 mg : 1.5 ml :: 500 mg : x ml
250 x = 750
x = 3 ml

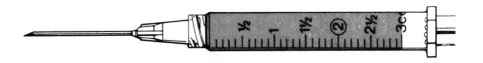

3. a. 2.5 ml

b. Sterile water for injection

c. Stable for 24 hours at room temperature; 96 hours if stored under refrigeration

d. 2 ml

$$\frac{\overset{2}{\cancel{660}\text{ mg}}}{\underset{1}{\cancel{330}\text{ mg}}} \times 1\text{ ml} = 2\text{ ml of Ancef}$$

330 mg : 1 ml :: 660 mg : x ml
330x = 660
x = 2 ml

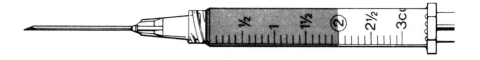

e. All of the solution, approximately 3 ml

$$\frac{1000\text{ mg}}{330\text{ mg}} \times 1\text{ ml} \approx 3\text{ ml}$$

330 mg : 1 ml :: 1000 mg : x ml
330 x = 1000
x ≈ 3 ml

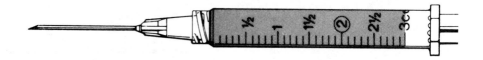

4. a. 50 to 100 ml

   b. Sodium chloride for injection or other intravenous solution listed in accompanying literature

   c. 24 hours at room temperature, 96 hours if refrigerated

5. a. Either 50 or 100 ml

   b. Sodium chloride for injection U.S.P. or dextrose injection U.S.P.

   c. Discard after 24 hours

   d. 500 mg to 1 g q6h

   e. 1 g in 100 ml, 10 g/ml
      1 g in 50 ml, 20 g/ml

      To mix Cefadyl you are given a choice of two strengths.

6. a. Add 1.8 ml diluent for IM use

   b. 250 to 500 mg IM q6h

   c. Give 2 ml SK ampicillin = N

      0.5 g = 500 mg

$$\frac{\overset{2}{\cancel{500}\text{ mg}}}{\underset{1}{\cancel{250}\text{ mg}}} \times 1\text{ ml} = 2\text{ ml}$$
of SK ampicillin-N

$$\frac{250\text{ mg}}{1\text{ ml}} :: \frac{500\text{ mg}}{x\text{ ml}}$$
$$250x = 500$$
$$x = 2\text{ ml}$$

7. a. 5 ml

   b. Water: shake well

   c. Discard after 14 days

   d. Give approximately 10 ml: two bottles

      0.25 g = 250 mg

$$\frac{\overset{2}{\cancel{250}\text{ mg}}}{\underset{1}{\cancel{125}\text{ mg}}} \times 5\text{ ml} = 10\text{ ml}$$

$$\frac{125\text{ mg}}{5\text{ ml}} :: \frac{250\text{ mg}}{x\text{ ml}}$$
$$125x = 1250$$
$$x = 10\text{ ml}$$

8. a. Add 2.5 ml sterile water for injection or 0.9% sodium chloride injection. Shake well. Protect from light

b. 3.0 ml (330 mg/ml)

c. Before reconstitution, store at controlled room temperature 59° to 86 °F (15° to 30 °C). After reconstitution, store in a refrigerator and use within 96 hours. If kept at room temperature, use within 24 hours

d. Give 2.3 ml of Kefzol every 6 hours

$$\frac{750 \text{ mg}}{330 \text{ mg}} \times 1 \text{ ml} = 2.27$$

$$\approx 2.3 \text{ ml}$$

$$330 \text{ mg}: 1 \text{ ml} :: 750 \text{ mg}: x \text{ ml}$$

$$\frac{330 \text{ mg}}{1 \text{ ml}} :: \frac{750 \text{ mg}}{x \text{ ml}}$$

$$330x = 750$$

$$x = 2.27 \approx 2.3 \text{ ml}$$

9. a. There are two strengths you could use:

    10 ml diluent   *OR*   4 ml diluent

b. Two strengths:

    10 ml = 100,000 U/ml   *OR*   4 ml = 250,000 U/ml

c. Using the dosage strength 100,000 U/ml, administer 2 ml of penicillin

$$\frac{200,000 \text{ U}}{100,000 \text{ U}} \times 1 \text{ ml} = 2 \text{ ml}$$

$$\frac{100,000 \text{ U}}{1 \text{ ml}} :: \frac{200,000 \text{ U}}{x \text{ ml}}$$

$$100,000x = 200,000$$

$$x = 2 \text{ ml}$$

Using the dosage strength 250,000 U/ml, administer 0.8 ml of penicillin

$$\frac{\overset{4}{\cancel{200,000}} \text{ U}}{\underset{5}{\cancel{250,000}} \text{ U}} \times 1 \text{ ml} = \frac{4}{5}$$

$$= 0.8 \text{ ml}$$

$$\frac{250,000 \text{ U}}{1 \text{ ml}} :: \frac{200,000 \text{ U}}{x \text{ ml}}$$

$$250,000 \, x = 200,000$$

$$x = 0.8 \text{ ml}$$

If you were confused and used 10 or 4 ml to work your problem, look at the label again. this penicillin bottle contains 1 million units—it is a multidose vial. Roerig lists four ways this powdered drug can be reconstituted. The label lists four different amounts of diluent that you can choose from to make the dosage strength desired. The diluent column is headed ''ml diluent added.'' the second column is headed ''units per ml of solution.'' Once the solution is mixed, forget the diluent and look at the second column. In this problem you should have chosen 10 ml of diluent, which makes a solution with 100,000 U of penicillin per milliliter (100,000 U/ml). If you chose 4 ml of diluent, the resulting solution strength is 250,000 U/ml. This is no different from the other problems you have seen except that the manufacturer gives you a choice of four strengths rather than only one.

10. a. In this problem you can choose to use 4 ml of diluent, which will make a solution 250,000 U/ml, or add 1.8 ml of diluent to make a dosage strength of 500,000 U/ml.

If you use 4 ml diluent,

$$\frac{\overset{7}{\cancel{350,000}} \text{ U}}{\underset{5}{\cancel{250,000}} \text{ U}} \times 1 \text{ ml} = \frac{7}{5}$$

$$= 1.4 \text{ ml}$$

$$\frac{250,000 \text{ U}}{1 \text{ ml}} :: \frac{350,000 \text{ U}}{x \text{ ml}}$$

$$250,000x = 350,000$$

$$x = 1.4 \text{ ml}$$

Give 1.4 ml Pfizerpen.

If you use 1.8 ml diluent,

$$\frac{\overset{7}{\cancel{350,000}} \text{ U}}{\underset{10}{\cancel{500,000}} \text{ U}} \times 1 \text{ ml} = \frac{7}{10}$$

$$= 0.7 \text{ ml}$$

$$\frac{500,000 \text{ U}}{1 \text{ ml}} :: \frac{350,000 \text{ U}}{x \text{ ml}}$$

$$500,000x = 350,000$$

$$x = 0.7 \text{ ml}$$

Give 0.7 ml Pfizerpen.

8

Pediatric Dosage

OBJECTIVES

After completing this chapter, the student will be able to:

1. State the difficulty in defining the appropriate child's dosage for drugs.
2. State Fried's rule.
3. Calculate children's dosage using Fried's rule.
4. State Young's rule.
5. Calculate children's dosage using Young's rule.
6. State Clark's rule.
7. Calculate children's dosage using Clark's rule.
8. Use the West nomogram for determining m² of skin surface of a child of normal height and weight.
9. Use the West nomogram to determine the body surface area (BSA) of a child not of average height or weight.
10. Calculate the surface area of a child using the formula

$$\frac{BSA\ m^2}{1.7\ m^2} \times \text{Adult dose} = \text{Pediatric dose}$$

11. Convert pounds to kilograms, and vice versa (lb $\rightleftharpoons$ kg).
12. Find dosages per body weight (using both kilograms of body weight and pounds of body weight).

Infants and children have special needs with regard to the appropriate dosage of medication. The growth rate of children for body weight, height, and physiological development varies greatly from child to child regardless of age. Many drug reference books do not state the pediatric dosage because the variance among children is so great. In fact, there is no standard dosage of medication for pediatric clients.

Until recently drug dosages were determined by research on adult subjects. Pediatric dosages were then extrapolated from this research. Today, large numbers of new, potentially dangerous drugs are becoming available yearly. They are still first tested on adult volunteers for dosage and side effects, and then tested to determine their effectiveness on patients having the condition they are designed to treat. Once they are determined to be effective and free of serious side effects, they are tested on children to determine their therapeutic value, the appropriate dosage, and any adverse side effects in children.

The dosage is usually established by determining the appropriate dosage per weight of the child (i.e., mg/kg/day or mg/lb/day in divided doses). Another method is to determine the dose per body surface area in square meters (BSA m^2). The BSA m^2 formula is used most frequently with drugs that are employed in the treatment of cancer (the antineoplastic drugs). Many adult doses are also based on these two formulas. You should use the dose per weight formula and BSA m^2 formula whenever the appropriate information is available. These two formulas will give you the most reliable index to the appropriate drug dose.

Regardless of the formula used to verify the appropriateness of drug dosage, you must assess the patient for his or her individual response to the drug. There is no substitute for astute assessment of the patient for drug effect, both for the therapeutic response and for any adverse side effects of the drug that might occur. *Remember:* the therapeutic range is often very small, especially in young infants. A small error in dosage calculation could lead to serious, even fatal results. You are legally responsible if a patient is harmed by the administration of an incorrect amount of drug. *Be safe, not sorry!*

FORMULAS BASED ON AGE

Fried's rule and Young's rule derive pediatric dosages from the adult dose on the basis of the child's age. These formulas do not take into consideration the wide variation in body size among children of the same age, therefore, they are only rarely used today. Clark's rule considers the child's weight, but here the dosage is derived from a formula that compares the child's weight to the weight of an average adult. A fraction of the adult's dose is then considered appropriate for the child. Clark's rule is probably more accurate than Fried's rule or Young's rule. It is sometimes used to check a child's dosage for accuracy when no information can be found in the drug reference books. These rules are never used to order a dosage, however, they are used to check the appropriateness of a dosage that has been ordered. They are discussed further and some examples of their use are given beginning on page 118.

FORMULAS BASED ON WEIGHT

Formulas based on weight and BSA are more accurate than those based on age. We first consider the formulas based on weight. Since you may need the weight in either kilograms or pounds, we need to review the conversion of pounds to kilograms, or kilograms to pounds.

Remember

$$2.2 \text{ lb} = 1 \text{ kg}$$

Therefore, to convert pounds to kilograms, divide the number of pounds by 2.2 or set up a ratio proportion:

$$36 \text{ lb} = x \text{ kg}$$
$$36 \text{ lb} \div 2.2 \text{ lb/kg} = 16.36 \text{ kg}$$

$$\frac{2.2 \text{ lb}}{1 \text{ kg}} = \frac{36 \text{ lb}}{x \text{ kg}}$$
$$2.2x = 36$$
$$x = 16.36 \text{ kg}$$

To convert kilograms to pounds, multiply the number of kilograms by 2.2 or set up a ratio and proportion:

$$14 \text{ kg} = x \text{ lb}$$
$$14 \text{ kg} \times 2.2 \text{ lb/kg} = 30.8 \text{ lb}$$

$$\frac{2.2 \text{ lb}}{1 \text{ kg}} = \frac{x \text{ lb}}{14 \text{ kg}}$$
$$x = 30.8 \text{ lb}$$

To determine whether you should multiply or divide, remember that a pound is a little more than twice as much as a kilogram. Therefore:

When converting from kilograms to pounds the answer should be more. When converting from pounds to kilograms the answer should be less.

Drug Dosage Calculated Per Milligram Per Child's Weight

The drug literature states the number of milligrams per weight (either pounds or kilograms) per day and per dose the patient should receive. The formula is

$$\left. \begin{array}{c} \text{mg/kg/day} \\ \text{or} \\ \text{mg/lb/day} \end{array} \right\} \text{ in } x \text{ number of equally divided doses}$$

Simply multiply the child's weight by the suggested dosage to obtain the amount of drug that can safely be administered per day and divide this by the number of doses per day.

Example 1

The physician has ordered Keflex 100 mg q6h (to be given every 6 hours) for a child weighing 12 kg. You want to be certain that the dosage is appropriate for this child.

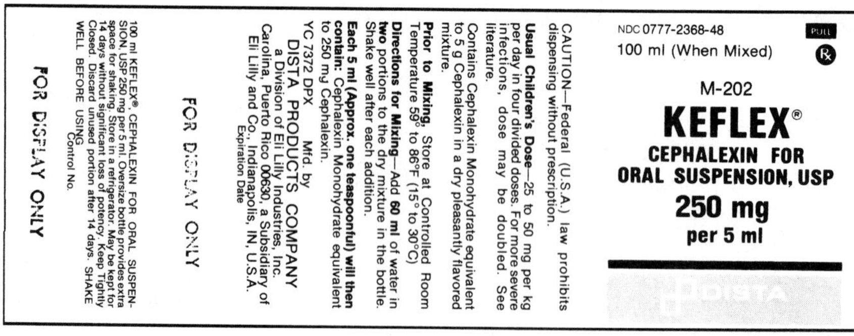

```
NDC 0777-2368-48                          PULL
100 ml (When Mixed)                        ℞

              M-202
KEFLEX®
CEPHALEXIN FOR
ORAL SUSPENSION, USP
  250 mg
  per 5 ml
```

(Label text, rotated:)

FOR DISPLAY ONLY

100 ml KEFLEX®. CEPHALEXIN FOR ORAL SUSPEN-
SION, USP 250 mg per 5 ml. Oversize bottle provides extra
space for shaking. Store in refrigerator. May be kept for
14 days without significant loss of potency. Keep Tightly
Closed. Discard unused portion after 14 days. SHAKE
WELL BEFORE USING.
              Control No.

YC 7372 DPX   Mfd. by
DISTA PRODUCTS COMPANY
a Division of Eli Lilly Industries, Inc.
Carolina, Puerto Rico 00630, a Subsidiary of
Eli Lilly and Co., Indianapolis, IN, U.S.A.
              Expiration Date

FOR DISPLAY ONLY

Directions for Mixing—Add **60 ml** of water in
two portions to the dry mixture in the bottle.
Shake well after each addition.
**Each 5 ml (Approx. one teaspoonful) will then
contain:** Cephalexin Monohydrate equivalent
to 250 mg Cephalexin.

Prior to Mixing, Store at Controlled Room
Temperature 59° to 86°F (15° to 30°C).

Contains Cephalexin Monohydrate equivalent
to 5 g Cephalexin in a dry pleasantly flavored
mixture.

Usual Children's Dose—25 to 50 mg per kg
per day in four divided doses. For more severe
infections, dose may be doubled. See
literature.

CAUTION—Federal (U.S.A.) law prohibits
dispensing without prescription.

Step 1: Read the Keflex medication label. (If the drug is not in the original package, refer to a good drug reference book that states the recommended child's dosage for Keflex.)

Under "Usual Children's Dose," the label states that 25 to 50 mg/ kg/day in four divided doses has been determined by drug research to be the usual therapeutic dose for a child. However, always remember that this is an average. It will not guarantee that the patient will not have an adverse reaction. You must always assess each patient's response to each drug.

Step 2: Substitute all known quantities into the formula.

$$\text{mg/dose} = \text{mg/kg/day} \div x \text{ number of equal doses}$$

The manufacturer has defined the safe range as 25 to 50 mg/kg/day in four divided doses. The child weighs 12 kg. Therefore,

$$25 \text{ mg/kg/day} \times 12 \text{ kg} = 300 \text{ mg/day} \div 4 \text{ doses} = 75 \text{ mg/dose}$$

Always check your math:

$$\textit{Proof:} \qquad 25\overline{)300} \quad \begin{array}{c} 12 \end{array}$$

This gives us the dosage for the lower limit (25 mg/kg/day) of the safe range. To determine the upper limit (50 mg/kg/day) we simply substitute 50 into the equation:

$$50 \text{ mg/kg/day} \times 12 \text{ kg} = 600 \text{ mg/day} \div 4 \text{ doses} = 150 \text{ mg/dose}$$

$$\textit{Proof:} \qquad 50\overline{)600} \quad \begin{array}{c} 12 \end{array}$$

The therapeutic range is therefore,

300 to 600 mg/day

or

75 to 150 mg/dose

Because 100 mg falls within the dosage range (75 to 150 mg), it will be safe to administer the ordered dosage. Remember always to observe the patient for drug effectiveness and for adverse side effects.

Step 3: Now that you have determined that the order falls within a safe therapeutic range, solve the dosage problem as you have learned to do in Chapter 4.

$$\frac{D}{H} \times V = G \qquad OR \qquad \frac{H}{V} :: \frac{D}{G} \qquad OR \qquad H:V::D:G$$

$$\frac{\overset{2}{\cancel{100}} \text{ mg}}{\underset{1}{\cancel{250}} \text{ mg}} \times \overset{1}{\cancel{5}} \text{ ml} = 2 \text{ ml} \qquad\qquad \frac{250 \text{ mg}}{5 \text{ ml}} :: \frac{100 \text{ mg}}{x \text{ ml}}$$

$$250x = 500$$
$$x = 2 \text{ ml}$$

Step 4: Check your arithmetic.
Substitute your answer for x and cross multiply.

$$250 \text{ mg} \div 5 \text{ ml} = 50 \text{ mg/ml} \qquad OR \qquad \frac{250 \text{ mg}}{5 \text{ ml}} :: \frac{100 \text{ mg}}{2 \text{ ml}}$$
$$50 \text{ mg/ml} \times 2 \text{ ml} = 100 \text{ mg} \qquad\qquad\qquad 250 \times 2 = 5 \times 100$$
$$500 = 500$$

Therefore, 2 ml is the correct dosage.

Step 5: Administer the medication on time following all safety guidelines that you have been taught.

Example 2

The physician ordered 250 mg of Cefaclor (Ceclor) tid (three times daily). The child has otitis media. The weight of the child is 39.6 lb. You are to administer the Cefaclor but first you want to check the appropriateness of the dosage ordered.

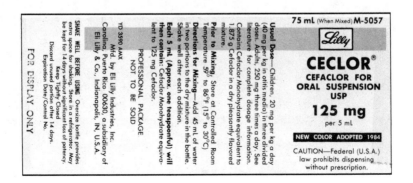

Question 1:
a. Read the Cefaclor label.
b. Substitute into the formula to determine the appropriateness of the dosage.

c. Is the physician's order appropriate? Why? or Why not?

Answer:
a. The Ceclor label gives the usual dose for children as 20 mg/kg/day (or 40 mg/kg/day for otitis media) in three divided doses.
b. Substitute into the formula.

$$mg/kg = \text{daily dosage divided into 3 doses/day}$$

In order to substitute into this formula the child's weight in pounds must first be converted to kilograms:

$$39.6 \text{ lg} \div 2.2 \text{ lb/kg} = 18 \text{ kg}$$

We can now substitute 18 kg into the formula:

$$40 \text{ mg/kg/day} \times 18 \text{ kg} = 720 \text{ mg/day} \div 3 \text{ doses} = 240 \text{ mg/dose}$$

c. The physician has ordered 250 mg/dose, which is more than the manufacturer recommends. You need to question this order.

Using the drug label, we now calculate the amount of Ceclor necessary to give Ceclor 240 mg.

$$\frac{D}{H} \times V = \text{dose}$$

$$\frac{240 \text{ mg}}{\underset{25}{\cancel{125} \text{ mg}}} \times \overset{1}{\cancel{5}} \text{ ml} = \frac{240}{25}$$

$$= 9.6 \text{ ml}$$

$$\frac{H}{V} :: \frac{D}{G} \text{ or } H:V::D:G$$

$$\frac{125 \text{ mg}}{5 \text{ ml}} :: \frac{240 \text{ mg}}{x \text{ ml}}$$

$$125x = 1200$$

$$x = \frac{1200}{125}$$

$$x = 9.6 \text{ ml}$$

Then check your arithmetic:

There are 25 mg/ml
25 mg/ml × 9.6 ml = 240 mg

$$\frac{125 \text{ mg}}{5 \text{ ml}} :: \frac{240 \text{ mg}}{9.6 \text{ ml}}$$

$$1200 = 1200$$

Administer 9.6 ml Ceclor.

Question 2: Calculate the amount of Ceclor necessary to give 250 mg.

Answer:

$$\frac{D}{H} \times V = G$$

$$\frac{2}{\cancel{250} \text{ mg}} \times 5 \text{ ml} = 10 \text{ ml}$$
$$\frac{\cancel{125} \text{ mg}}{1}$$

$$\frac{H}{V} :: \frac{D}{G}$$

$$\frac{125 \text{ mg}}{5 \text{ ml}} :: \frac{250 \text{ mg}}{x \text{ ml}}$$
$$125x = 1250$$
$$x = 10 \text{ ml}$$

Proof:

$$25 \text{ mg/ml} \times 10 \text{ ml} = 250 \text{ mg}$$

$$\frac{125 \text{ mg}}{5 \text{ ml}} = \frac{250 \text{ mg}}{10 \text{ ml}}$$
$$1250 = 1250$$

A 9.6 ml dose would be a difficult amount for a parent to measure. Ten milliliters equals 2 teaspoons. The physician probably ordered 250 mg in order that the parent could use a teaspoon to administer the drug at home. The difference between 240 mg and 250 mg is about 4 percent. Ten percent above the manufacturer's recommended dose is considered an acceptable amount. Four percent is well within this limit. Although 9.6 ml cannot be measured in a medicine glass, it could be measured in a 10 ml syringe. An oral medicine syringe may be purchased in a drugstore for home use.

Example 3

The physician ordered 70 mg doxycycline monohydrate (Vibramycin) for a 38-lb child on the first day of treatment. Is this an appropriate dose? Why or why not?

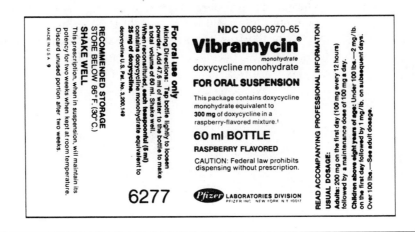

Step 1: The medication label states for children above 8 years of age: Under 100 lb, give 2 mg/lb on the first day followed by 1 mg/lb on subsequent days.

Step 2: Substitute into the formula.

$$2 \text{ mg/lb/day} \times 38 \text{ lb} = 76 \text{ mg/day}$$

The physician's order is less than the manufacturer recommendation. Question this order.

Exercises: Formulas Based on Dose per Weight Formula

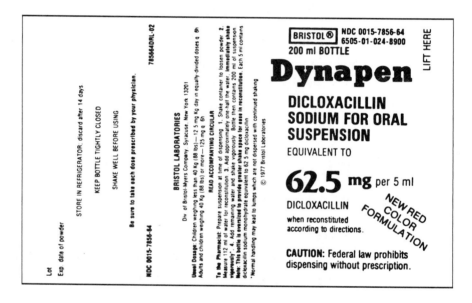

1. The physician ordered Dynapen 100 mg every 6 hours to be given by mouth to a child whose weight is 32 kg.
   a. Using the drug manufacturer's recommendation given on the label, is the dose 100 mg appropriate for a child weighing 32 kg? Explain your answer.

   b. How many milliliters of Dynapen will be needed to administer 100 mg of drug?

2. The physician ordered Dynapen 125 mg every 6 hours to be given by mouth to a child whose weight is 36 kg. Is this dose appropriate for a child weighing 36 kg? Explain your answer.

3. The physician ordered amikacin sulfate, 170 mg IV every 12 hours, for a child who weighs 50 lb.

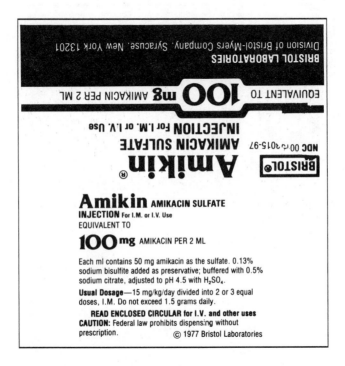

a. Using the drug manufacturer's recommendation given on the label, how much drug should a child who weighs 50 lb receive per day? Per dose?

b. Is the doctor's order appropriate for a 50 lb child? Explain your answer.

c. How many milliliters of amikacin sulfate should be put in the IV to be administered every 8 hours?

4. The physician ordered Vibramycin 80 mg every 12 hours for 24 hours. The child weighs 80 lb.

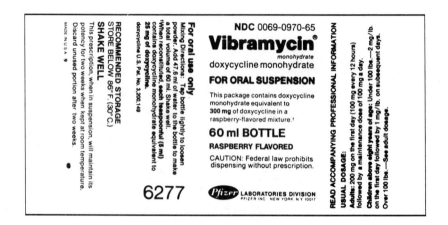

a. Using the manufacturer's recommendation given on the label, how much Vibramycin should a child who weighs 80 lb receive on the first day that the drug is given?

b. Is the doctor's order appropriate for an 80-lb child? Explain your answer.

c. How many milliliters of Vibramycin should be given?

5. The physician ordered Keflex 70 mg po qid (by mouth four times a day).
   a. Using the Keflex drug label, determine if the dosage ordered is appropriate. The child weighs 6.25 kg.

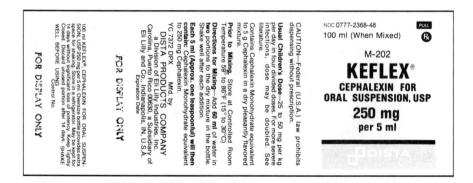

b. Calculate the amount of Keflex needed to administer 70 mg of drug.

Answers

1. a. Yes, the manufacturer recommends 12.5 mg/kg/day for children weighing less than 40 kg (88 lb):

$$12.5 \text{ mg/kg/day} \times 32 \text{ kg} = 400 \text{ mg/day of Dynapen}$$
$$400 \text{ mg} \div 4 \text{ doses} = 100 \text{ mg/dose of Dynapen}$$

   b.

$$\frac{100 \text{ mg}}{62.5 \text{ mg}} \times 5 \text{ ml} = 8 \text{ ml}$$

   $62.5 \text{ mg} : 5 \text{ ml} :: 100 \text{ mg} : x \text{ ml}$
   $62.5x = 500$
   $x = 8 \text{ ml}$

2. No, it is more than the manufacturer recommends. Question this order.

$$12.5 \text{ mg/kg/day} \times 36 \text{ kg} = 450 \text{ mg/day of Dynapen}$$
$$450 \text{ mg} \div 4 \text{ doses} = 112.5 \text{ mg/dose of Dynapen}$$

3. a. First convert the pounds to kilograms:

$$
\begin{array}{r}
22.72 \text{ kg} \\
2.2 \text{ kg} \overline{)50.0.0 \text{ lb}} \\
\underline{44} \\
60 \\
\underline{44} \\
160 \\
\underline{154} \\
60 \\
\underline{44}
\end{array}
$$

Then substitute 22.72 kg into the formula:

$$15 \text{ mg/kg/day} \times 22.72 \text{ kg} = 340.8 \text{ mg/day amikacin sulfate}$$

$$340.8 \text{ mg} \div 2 \text{ doses} = 170.4 \text{ or } 170 \text{ mg/dose amikacin sulfate}$$

b. Yes, the recommended dose for a child weighing 50 lb is 170 mg.

c. $\dfrac{170 \text{ mg}}{100 \text{ mg}} \times 2 \text{ ml} = \dfrac{340}{100} \text{ ml}$ $100 \text{ mg} : 2 \text{ ml} :: 170 \text{ mg} : x \text{ ml}$

$\qquad\qquad\qquad\qquad = 3.4 \text{ ml of Amikacin}$ $100x = 340$

$\qquad\qquad\qquad\qquad\qquad\qquad\qquad\qquad\qquad\qquad x = 3.4 \text{ ml}$

4. a. $\qquad\qquad 2 \text{ mg/lb/day} \times 80 \text{ lb} = 160 \text{ mg/day of Vibramycin}$

$\qquad\qquad\qquad 160 \div 2 \text{ doses} = 80 \text{ mg of Vibramycin}$

b. Yes, the dosage ordered, 80 mg, is the recommended amount.

c. $\dfrac{\overset{16}{\cancel{80} \text{ mg}}}{\underset{5}{\cancel{25} \text{ mg}}} \times \overset{1}{\cancel{5}} \text{ ml} = 16 \text{ ml of Vibramycin}$ $\dfrac{25 \text{ mg}}{5 \text{ ml}} :: \dfrac{80 \text{ mg}}{x \text{ ml}}$

$\qquad\qquad\qquad\qquad\qquad\qquad\qquad\qquad\qquad\qquad 25x = 400$

$\qquad\qquad\qquad\qquad\qquad\qquad\qquad\qquad\qquad\qquad\quad x = 16 \text{ ml}$

5. a. Yes, the dose ordered is within the appropriate dosage range.

$$25 \text{ mg/kg/day} \times 6.25 \text{ kg} = 156.25 \text{ mg} \div 4 \text{ doses}$$

$$= 39.06 \approx 39 \text{ mg of Keflex/dose}$$

$$50 \text{ mg/kg/day} \times 6.25 \text{ kg} = 312.5 \div 4 \text{ doses}$$

$$= 78.12 \approx 78 \text{ mg of Keflex/dose}$$

b. $\dfrac{\overset{7}{\cancel{70} \text{ mg}}}{\underset{\underset{5}{\cancel{25}}}{\cancel{250} \text{ mg}}} \times \overset{1}{\cancel{5}} \text{ ml} = \dfrac{7}{5} \text{ ml}$ $\dfrac{250 \text{ mg}}{5 \text{ ml}} :: \dfrac{70 \text{ mg}}{x \text{ ml}}$

$\qquad\qquad\qquad\qquad\qquad\qquad\qquad\qquad 250x = 350$

$\qquad\qquad\qquad\qquad = 1.4 \text{ ml of Keflex} \qquad\qquad x = 1.4 \text{ ml}$

FORMULAS BASED ON BODY SURFACE AREA

One of the more accurate methods to determine pediatric dosages is based on body surface area (BSA). The use of both height and weight correlates closely to the child's physiologic development. This method is not appropriate for very small infants.

The West nomogram, shown on page 110, uses both height and weight to determine the BSA of a child. Other nomograms may also be used to determine the BSA of children. There are also nomograms to determine the BSA of adults.

Note: When using the West nomogram, be aware that the scales vary as they ascend. Be sure to figure the amount each line represents before reading the scale value.

To determine the BSA of a child of normal height and weight, use the scale within the boxed insert on the West nomogram.

1. Place a straight edge on the child's weight in pounds.
2. Read the surface area on the adjacent scale.

Example 1

What is the surface area of a child of normal height and weight weighing 10 lb?

Using the boxed insert, we align 10 lb with the BSA of 0.27 m². (See nomogram on page 110.)

To determine the BSA in square meters (m²) for a child whose weight and height are not within normal limits:

1. Weigh the child in either pounds or kilograms.
2. Measure the child in either centimeters or inches.
3. Place a straight edge (ruler or piece of paper) from the height of the child on the left-hand scale to the weight of the child on the right-hand scale.
4. Read the surface area scale where the line between the height and weight intersects the surface area scale.

Example 2

What is the BSA for a child weighing 15 kg and 86 cm tall? As is shown in the nomogram on page 110, drawing a line between 15 kg and 86 cm, we find

$$BSA = 0.62 \text{ m}^2$$

Once the BSA has been determined, the pediatric dose can be determined from the adult dose using the following formula:

$$\frac{\text{Surface area (m}^2) \times \text{Adult dose}}{1.7 \text{ m}^2} = \text{Pediatric dose}$$

(Although 1.73 m² may also be used, this book will use 1.7 m².) Using the BSA found in example 2, we will now calculate the pediatric dose of a drug when the adult dose is 325 mg:

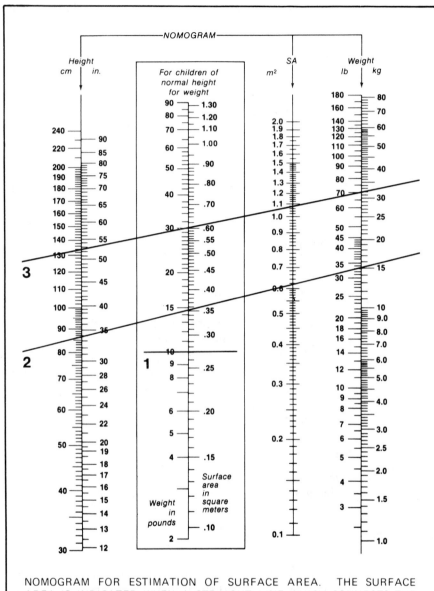

West nomogram showing answers to examples 1, 2, and 3. (*Adapted from Behrman, R. & Vaughan, V.: Nelson Textbook of Pediatrics, 13th Ed. Philadelphia, W. B. Saunders Co., 1987.*)

$$\frac{SA(m^2) \times Adult\ dose}{1.7\ m^2} = Pediatric\ dose$$

$$\frac{0.62\ m^2}{1.7\ m^2} \times 325\ mg = \frac{201.5}{1.7}\ mg$$

$$= 118.529\ mg \approx 118.53\ mg$$

The dosage for certain drugs is given in milligrams per square meter (mg/m²). To determine the dosage to give, you multiply the number of milligrams by the value of m².

Example 3

What is the recommended dose of acyclovir (Zovirax) for a child weighing 32 kg whose height is 134 cm if the dosage is 250 mg/m² tid?

Step 1: First determine BSA using the West nomogram:

$$BSA = 1.08\ m^2$$

Step 2: Substitute into the formula:

$$250\ mg \times 1.08\ m^2 = 270\ mg/dose$$
$$270\ mg/dose \times 3\ doses/day = 810\ mg/day$$

Exercises: Body Surface Area

Use the nomogram on page 112 to determine the BSA for problems 1 through 5. Carry out all answers to the nearest hundredth.

1. The average intravenous dose of doxorubicin (Adriamycin) for a child is 30 mg/m². Using the BSA formula, calculate the dosage for a child whose weight is 50 kg and height is 160 cm.

2. The physician orders vincristine (Oncovin) 1.5 mg IV once a week for a child whose weight is 20 kg and height is 110 cm. The recommended dose for children is 1.5 to 2 mg/m². Is this dose appropriate?

3. The physician ordered acyclovir (Zovirax) 130 mg for a child whose weight is 28 lb and height is 34 in. Is this dose appropriate for this child if the recommended dose is 250 mg/m²/dose or 750 mg/m²/day?

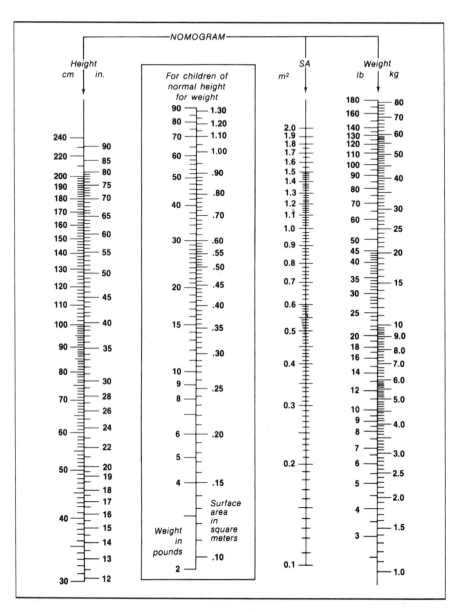

Use to determine the BSA (m²) for problems 1 to 5

4. The adult dosage of a drug is 40 mg/dose. Determine the BSA and calculate the dosage for a child weighing 30 lb and 36 in tall.

5. The average intravenous dose of Adriamycin for a child is 30 mg/m². Determine the BSA and calculate the dosage for a child weighing 25 kg and 100 cm tall.

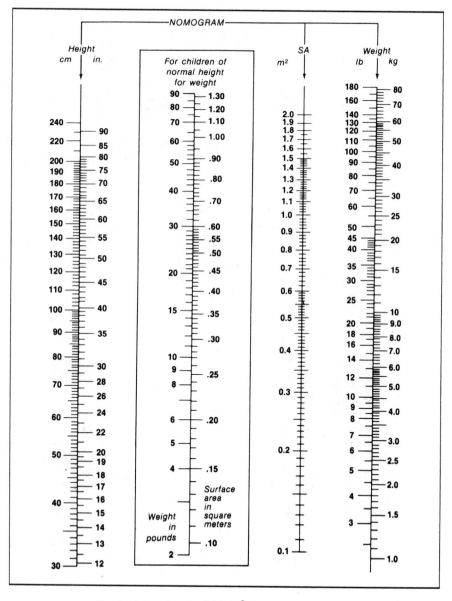

Use to determine the BSA (m²) for problems 6 to 10.

Use the West nomogram to determine the BSA of the following children of normal height and weight. Mark your answers on the nomogram on page 113.

6. 44 lb = _____ m²

7. 36 lb = _____ m²

8. 85 lb = _____ m²

9.   5 lb = _____ m²

10. 10 lb = _____ m²

Answers: Body Surface Area

Refer to page 115 for the West nomogram used to determine the BSA in problems 1 through 3, page 116 for problems 4 and 5, and page 117 for problems 6 through 10.

1. We determine the BSA by drawing a straight line from 50 kg to 160 cm on the West nomogram. The BSA is 1.5 m². We then substitute this value into the following equation in order to determine the dosage appropriate for this child:

$$30 \text{ mg/m}^2 \times 1.5 \text{ m}^2 = 45.0 \text{ mg}$$

2. The BSA is 0.78 m². The dosage range is therefore

$$1.5 \text{ mg/m}^2 \times 0.78 \text{ m}^2 = 1.17 \text{ mg}$$
$$2 \text{ mg/m}^2 \times 0.78 \text{ m}^2 = 1.56 \text{ mg}$$

The dose ordered (1.5 mg/m²) is in the appropriate range (i.e.,: 1.17 to 1.56 mg).

3. BSA = 0.565 m²

$$250 \text{ mg/m}^2/\text{dose} \times 0.565 \text{ m}^2 = 141.25 \text{ mg/dose}$$

The dosage ordered is insufficient. Question this order.

4. BSA = 0.6 m²

$$\frac{\text{SA m}^2}{1.7 \text{ m}^2} \times \text{Adult dose} = \text{Pediatric dose}$$

$$\frac{0.6 \text{ m}^2}{1.7 \text{ m}^2} \times 40 \text{ mg} = \frac{24}{1.7} = 14.117 \text{ mg} \approx 14.12 \text{ mg}$$

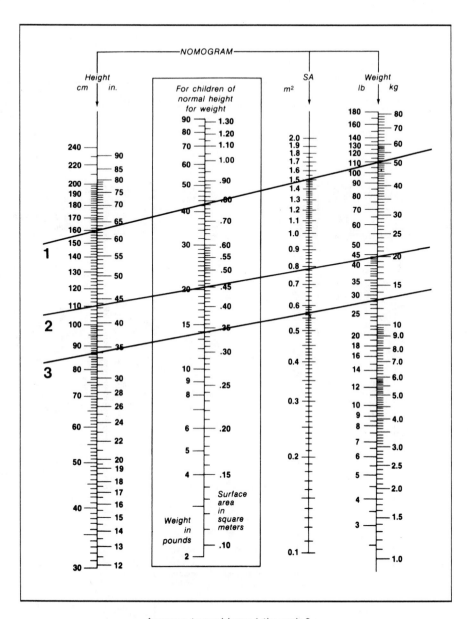

---NOMOGRAM---

Height
cm   in.

SA
m²

Weight
lb   kg

For children of
normal height
for weight

Weight
in
pounds

Surface
area
in
square
meters

Answers to problems 1 through 3.

5. BSA = 0.86 m²

$$30 \text{ mg/m}^2 \times 0.86 \text{ m}^2 = 25.8 \text{ mg}$$

6. 44 lb = $\underline{\text{0.8 m}^2}$

7. 36 lb = $\underline{\text{0.68 m}^2}$

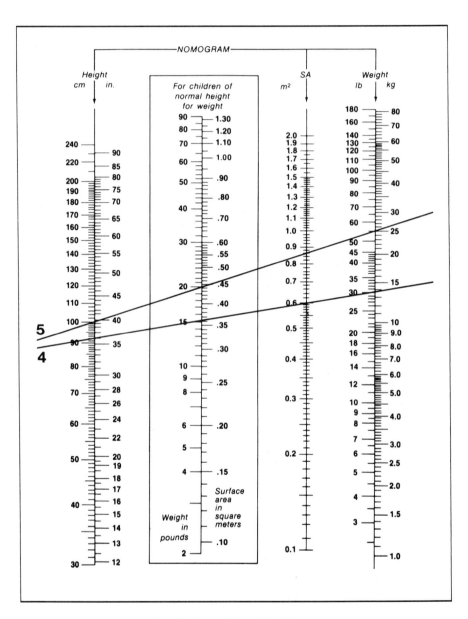

Answers to problems 4 and 5.

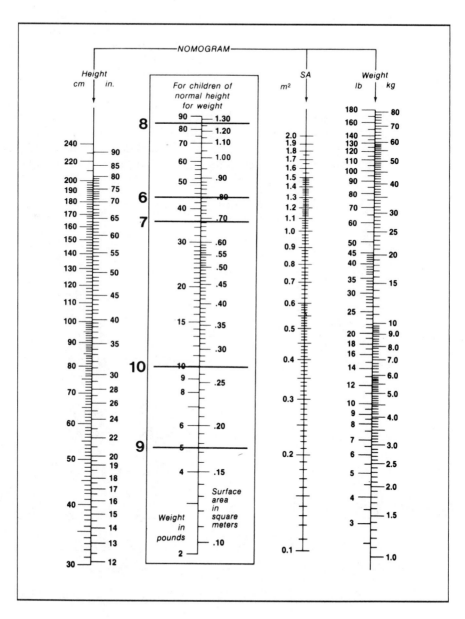

Answers to problems 6 through 10.

    8. 85 lb = <u> 1.27 m^2 </u>

    9.   5 lb = <u> 0.175 m^2 </u>

  10. 10 lb = <u> 0.27 m^2 </u>

CLARK'S RULE

Clark's rule determines the drug dosage for infants and children based upon body weight. It may be used to confirm the safety of a physician's order but is never used to prescribe the child's actual dose. Clark's rule provides a more accurate approximation for children's dosages than formulas based on age.

$$\frac{\text{Child's weight (lb)}}{150 \text{ lb}} \times \text{Adult dose} = \text{Pediatric dose}$$

(this is an average adult weight.)

Example

How much Keflin should a 20-lb child receive if the adult dose is 500 mg?

Substitute into the formula.

$$\frac{\text{Child's weight}}{150 \text{ lb}} \times \text{Adult dose} = \text{Pediatric dose}$$

$$\frac{\overset{2}{\cancel{20} \text{ lb}}}{\underset{15}{\cancel{150} \text{ lb}}} \times 500 \text{ mg} = \frac{1000}{15} = 66.666 \approx 66.67 \text{ mg}$$

Exercises: Clark's Rule

Solve the following problems using Clark's rule. Round your answer to the nearest hundredth.

1. How much Minocin should be given to a 58-lb child if the adult dose is 100 mg?

2. How much methicillin should be given to a 36-lb child if the adult dose is 1000 mg?

3. How much Tylenol should be given to a child weighing 21 lb if the adult dose is 300 to 650 mg?

4. How much Aldomet should a 60-lb child receive if the adult dose is 500 mg?

5. How much Compazine should a 54-lb child receive if the adult dose is 10 mg?

Answers: Clark's Rule

1.
$$\frac{58 \text{ lb}}{\underset{3}{\cancel{150} \text{ lb}}} \times \overset{2}{\cancel{100}} \text{ mg} = \frac{116}{3} = 38.666 \approx 38.67 \text{ mg Minocin}$$

2.
$$\frac{36 \text{ lb}}{\underset{3}{\cancel{150} \text{ lb}}} \times \overset{20}{\cancel{1000}} \text{ mg} = \frac{720}{3} = 240 \text{ mg methicillin}$$

3.
$$\frac{21 \text{ lb}}{\underset{1}{\cancel{150} \text{ lb}}} \times \overset{2}{\cancel{300}} \text{ mg} = 42 \text{ mg Tylenol}$$

$$\frac{\overset{7}{\cancel{21}} \text{ lb}}{\underset{1}{\cancel{150} \text{ lb}}} \times \overset{13}{\cancel{650}} \text{ mg} = 91 \text{ mg Tylenol}$$

4.
$$\frac{\overset{6}{\cancel{60}}\text{lb}}{\underset{15}{\cancel{150}\text{lb}}} \times 500 \text{ mg} = \frac{3000}{15} = 200 \text{ mg Aldomet}$$

5.
$$\frac{54 \text{ lb}}{\underset{15}{\cancel{150}\text{lb}}} \times \overset{1}{\cancel{10}} \text{ mg} = \frac{54}{15} = 3.6 \text{ mg Compazine}$$

FRIED'S RULE

Fried's rule is used to determine the dosage for infants less than 1 year of age. It should not be used to calculate dosages but can be used to check the physician's order. Question any dosage that does not agree.

$$\frac{\text{Age of infant (months)}}{150 \text{ lb}} \times \text{Adult dose} = \text{Estimated safe dose for an infant}$$

Example

The adult dose of a certain drug is 100 mg. Determine the dose for an 8-month-old infant using Fried's rule.

$$\frac{8 \text{ mo}}{\underset{3}{\cancel{150}}} \times \overset{2}{\cancel{100}} \text{ mg} = \frac{16}{3} = 5\frac{1}{3} \text{ mg or } 5.33 \text{ mg}$$

Exercises: Fried's Rule

1. The average adult dose of Drug A is 1000 mg. Use Fried's rule to determine an appropriate dose for a 4-month-old infant.

2. The average adult dose of Drug B is 10 mg. What is an appropriate dose for a 5-month-old infant?

3. The average adult dose of Drug C is 0.4 mg. What is an appropriate dose for an 8-month-old infant?

Answers: Fried's Rule

1.
$$\frac{\text{Age of infant in months}}{150} \times \text{Adult dose} = \text{Infant dose}$$

$$\frac{4 \text{ mo}}{\underset{3}{\cancel{150} \text{ lb}}} \times \overset{20}{\cancel{1000}} \text{mg} = \frac{80}{3} = 26.666 \approx 26.67 \text{ mg Drug A}$$

2.
$$\frac{\overset{1}{\cancel{8} \text{ mo}}}{\underset{\underset{3}{\cancel{15}}}{\cancel{150} \text{ lb}}} \times \overset{1}{\cancel{10}} \text{mg} = \frac{1}{3} = 0.333 \approx 0.33 \text{ mg Drug B}$$

3.
$$\frac{8 \text{ mo}}{150 \text{ lb}} \times 0.4 \text{ mg} = \frac{3.2}{150} = 0.02 \text{ mg Drug C}$$

YOUNG'S RULE

Young's rule is used to determine the dose for a child between 1 and 12 years of age. It should not be used to calculate dosages but can be used to check the physician's order. Question any dosage that does not agree.

$$\frac{\text{Age of child (yr)}}{\text{Age of child (yr)} + 12} \times \text{Adult dose} = \text{Estimated safe dose for a child}$$

Example

The adult dose for a drug is 150 mg. Determine the dose of the drug for a 5-year-old child.

$$\frac{5}{5 + 12} \times 150 \text{ mg} = \text{Child's dose}$$

$$\frac{5}{17} \times 150 = \frac{750}{17} = 44.117 \approx 44.12 \text{ mg}$$

Exercises: Young's Rule

1. The average adult dose for Drug A is 200 mg. What is an appropriate dose for a 9-year-old child?

2. The average adult dose for Drug B is 25 mg. What is an appropriate dose for an 11-year-old child?

3. The average adult dose for Drug C is 4 mg. What is an appropriate dose for a 5-year-old child?

Answers: Young's Rule

1. $$\frac{\text{Age of child (yr)}}{\text{Age of child (yr) } + \text{ 12}} \times \text{Adult dose} = \text{Child's dose}$$

$$\frac{9}{9 + 12} \times 200 \text{ mg} = \frac{\overset{3}{\cancel{9}}}{\underset{7}{\cancel{21}}} \times 200$$

$$= \frac{600}{7} = 85.714 \approx 85.71 \text{ mg Drug A}$$

2. $$\frac{11}{11 + 12} \times 25 \text{ mg} = \frac{11}{23} \times 25$$

$$= \frac{275}{23} = 11.956 \approx 11.96 \text{ mg Drug B}$$

3. $$\frac{5}{5 + 12} \times 4 \text{ mg} = \frac{5}{17} \times 4 = \frac{20}{17} \text{ mg}$$

$$= 1.176 \text{ mg} \approx 1.18 \text{ mg Drug C}$$

PROBLEMS: PEDIATRIC DOSAGE

Carry out your answers to the nearest hundredth place.

Clark's Rule

1. The physician ordered aspirin 150 mg for a 40-lb child. The adult dose for aspirin is 300 to 600 mg. How much aspirin is safe for a 40-lb child? Is the dose ordered within the safe range?

2. The physician ordered 25 mg of meperidine hydrochloride for a 50-lb child preoperatively. Is this a safe dose? The adult dose is 25 to 100 mg.

3. The physician ordered 50 mg Vistaril for a 75-lb boy. The adult dose is 100 mg. Is the dose ordered within the safe range?

4. The physician ordered 120,000 U Bicillin for a 30-lb child. The adult dose is 600,000 U. Is the dose ordered within the safe range?

Young's Rule

5. The average adult dose of a drug is 4 g. What would be an appropriate dose of the drug for a 10-year-old child?

6. The average adult dose of a drug is 150 mg. What would be an appropriate dose for a 6-year-old child?

Fried's Rule

7. The average adult dose of a drug is 500 mg. What would be an appropriate dose of the drug for a 6-month-old infant?

8. The average adult dose of a drug is 250 mg. What would be an appropriate dose of the drug for a 3-month-old infant?

Body Surface Area

Use the nomogram on page 128 to find the BSAs in questions 9 through 12.

9. a. Determine the BSA of a child of normal height weighing 22 lb.

   b. The adult dose of a drug is 4 g. What is an appropriate dose for this child?

10. a. Determine the BSA of a child weighing 40 kg who is 110 cm tall.

    b. The adult dose of Unipen is 500 mg. Determine the dose of Unipen appropriate for this child.

11. a. Determine the BSA of a 6-lb infant of normal height.

    b. What is the appropriate dose for this child if the adult dose of gentamicin is 250 mg q6h?

12. a. Determine the BSA of a child 85 cm tall, weighing 30 lb.

    b. If the adult dose of a drug is 300 mcg, what is the appropriate dose for this child?

Dosage per Weight

13. A 40-lb child is to receive Unipen. The usual pediatric dose is 25 to 50 mg/kg/day in four divided doses. What is the appropriate dosage range for this child?

14. The pediatric dose of gentamicin is 3 to 6 mg/kg/day in divided doses. Determine the dosage range when the infant weighs 6 kg.

15. The pediatric dose of kanamycin is 7.5 to 15 mg/kg/day in divided doses. How much drug will a child weighing 45 kg receive per day? How much per dose if the drug is given in four equal doses?

16. The pediatric dose of Dilantin is 4 to 8 mg/kg/day in divided doses. How much drug will a child weighing 60 lb receive?

ANSWERS: PEDIATRIC DOSAGE

Clark's Rule

1. $$\frac{\text{Child's weight}}{\text{Average adult weight}} \times \text{Adult dose} = \text{Estimated pediatric dose}$$

$$\frac{\overset{4}{\cancel{40}}\text{ lb}}{\underset{15}{\cancel{150}}\text{ lb}} \times \overset{20}{\cancel{300}}\text{ mg} = 80 \text{ mg}$$

$$\frac{40}{\cancel{150}} \times \overset{4}{\cancel{600}}\text{ mg} = 160 \text{ mg}$$

The dose of aspirin is within the safe range.

2.

$$\frac{\overset{1}{\cancel{50}\text{ lb}}}{\underset{3}{\cancel{150}\text{ lb}}} \times 25 \text{ mg} = \frac{25}{3} \approx 8.33 \text{ mg}$$

$$\frac{\overset{1}{\cancel{50}\text{ lb}}}{\underset{3}{\cancel{150}\text{ lb}}} \times 100 \text{ mg} = \frac{100}{3} \approx 33.33 \text{ mg}$$

The estimated range for a 50-lb child is 8.3 to 33.3 mg. The order is within this range.

3.

$$\frac{75 \text{ lb}}{\underset{3}{\cancel{150}\text{ lb}}} \times \overset{2}{\cancel{100}} \text{ mg} = \frac{150}{3} = 50 \text{ mg}$$

The dose is safe.

4.

$$\frac{30}{\underset{1}{\cancel{150}}} \times \overset{4000}{\cancel{600,000}} \text{ U} = 120,000 \text{ U}$$

The dose ordered is in the safe range.

Young's Rule

5. $$\frac{\text{Age of child (yr)}}{\text{Age of child (yr)} + 12} \times \text{Adult dose} = \text{Estimated pediatric dose}$$

$$\frac{10}{10 + 12} \times 4 \text{ g} = \frac{40}{22} = 1.818 \text{ g} \approx 1.82 \text{ g}$$

6. $$\frac{6}{6 + 12} \times 150 \text{ mg} = \frac{900}{18} = 50 \text{ mg}$$

Fried's Rule

7. $$\frac{\text{Infant's age (mo)}}{150 \text{ lb}} \times \text{Adult dose} = \text{Estimated infant dose}$$

$$\frac{6 \text{ mo}}{150 \text{ lb}} \times 500 \text{ mg} = \frac{3000}{150} = 20 \text{ mg}$$

8. $$\frac{3 \text{ mo}}{150 \text{ lb}} \times 250 \text{ mg} = \frac{750}{150} = 5 \text{ mg}$$

Body Surface Area

    9. a. 0.47 m^2

        b. $\dfrac{\text{Surface area (m}^2)}{1.7 \text{ m}^2} \times \text{Adult dose} = \text{Pediatric dose}$

$$\frac{0.47 \text{ m}^2}{1.7 \text{ m}^2} \times 4 \text{ g} = \frac{1.88}{1.7} = 1.105 \text{ g} \approx 1.11 \text{ g}$$

  10. a. 1.14 m^2

        b. $\dfrac{1.14 \text{ m}^2}{1.7 \text{ m}^2} \times 500 \text{ mg} = \dfrac{570}{1.7} = 335.294 \text{ mg} \approx 335.29 \text{ g}$

  11. a. 0.2 m^2

        b. $\dfrac{0.2 \text{ m}^2}{1.7 \text{ m}^2} \times 250 \text{ mg} = \dfrac{50}{1.7} = 29.411 \text{ mg} \approx 29.41 \text{ mg}$

  12. a. 0.58 m^2

        b. $\dfrac{0.58 \text{ m}^2}{1.7 \text{ m}^2} \times 300 \text{ mcg} = \dfrac{174}{1.7} = 102.352 \text{ mcg} \approx 102.35 \text{ mcg}$

Dosage Per Weight

  13. Convert pounds to kilograms:

$$40 \text{ lb} \div 2.2 \text{ lb/kg} = 18.181 \text{ kg} \approx 18.18 \text{ kg}$$

$$18.18 \text{ kg} \times 25 \text{ mg/kg/day} = 454.5 \text{ mg/day} \div 4 \text{ doses/day}$$
$$= 113.625 \approx 113.63 \text{ mg/dose}$$

$$18.18 \text{ kg} \times 50 \text{ mg/kg/day} = 909.0 \text{ mg/day} \div 4 \text{ doses/day}$$
$$= 227.25 \text{ mg/dose}$$

Range: 454.5 to 909.0 mg/day or 113.63 to 227.25 mg/dose

  14.

$$6 \text{ kg} \times 3 \text{ mg/kg/day} = 18 \text{ mg/day}$$

$$6 \text{ kg} \times 6 \text{ mg/kg/day} = 36 \text{ mg/day}$$

Range: 18 to 36 mg/day

  15. $45 \text{ kg} \times 7.5 \text{ mg/kg/day} = 337.5 \text{ mg/day} \div 4 \text{ doses/day}$
$$= 84.375 \approx 84.38 \text{ mg/dose}$$

$$45 \text{ kg} \times 15 \text{ mg/kg/day} = 675 \text{ mg/day} \div 4 \text{ doses/day}$$
$$= 168.75 \text{ mg/dose}$$

Range: 337.5 to 675 mg/day or 84.38 to 168.75 mg/dose

16.   60 lb. ÷ 2.2 lb/kg = 27.272 kg ≈ 27.27 kg

27.27 kg × 4 mg/kg/day = 109.08 mg/day

27.27 kg × 8 mg/kg/day = 218.16 mg/day

Range: 109.08 to 218.16 mg/day

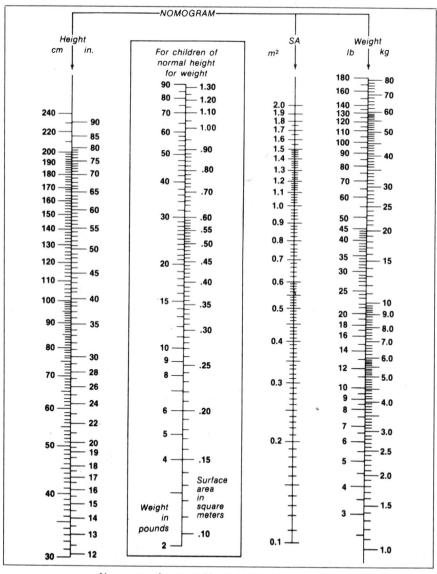

Nomogram for use with problems 9 through 12.

9

Intravenous Fluid Rate Calculation

OBJECTIVES

After completing this chapter, the student will be able to:

1. Calculate the 1-hour volume from a 24-hour volume of IV fluid.
2. Use the formula given to calculate the number of drops per minute needed to administer a given volume of intravenous fluid. Use an administration set with a drop factor of 10, 15, 20, or 60 drops per milliliter (gtt/ml).
3. Calculate the flow rate of an IV administration set using a drop factor other than 10, 15, 20, or 60 gtt/ml.
4. Calculate the flow rate of IV medications to be administered in small volumes of intravenous fluid.
5. Calculate the volume of intravenous fluid containing a specified amount of drug to be administered in 1 hour.
6. State the purpose of volume control sets (i.e., Buretrol).
7. Determine the amount of medication and fluid to put into the volume control set.
8. Calculate the infusion rate of the volume control set with medication added.
9. Knowing the amount of drug to be administered per hour, calculate the flow rate.
10. Calculate the infusion rate, in drops per minute, needed to administer an ordered amount of drug per hour.
11. Knowing the amount of drug to be administered per minute, calculate the 1-minute volume that will result.
12. Calculate the infusion rate needed to administer the ordered amount of drug per minute.
13. Adjust the IV flow rate for IVs running off schedule.

INTRAVENOUS INFUSIONS

The use of intravenous (IV) infusions has increased dramatically in recent years. It is very important to be able to regulate the flow of IV fluids carefully because of the dangers inherent in parenteral fluid administration. The number of medications given intravenously has also increased drastically. This chapter provides the mathematical formulas necessary for IV administration.

The flow rate of IV fluids is controlled by calibrated administration sets. Each brand of IV administration set has a calculated rate of flow, for example, 10, 13, 15, 20, or 60 drops per milliliter (gtt/ml). This rate of flow is termed the *drop factor* and is listed on the carton containing the IV set.

The physician will order the amount of IV fluid to be infused per day, per hour, or sometimes, even the flow rate (drops per minute).

Memorize the formulas that follow—you will use them frequently.

LARGE-VOLUME IV ADMINISTRATION

Formula:

$$\frac{\text{Drop factor}}{\text{Time}} \times \text{Volume} = \text{Flow rate}$$

Drop factor is the calibrated rate of flow of the administration set. This rate (i.e., 10 or 15 gtt/ml) is listed on the box containing the IV tubing.
Time in the formula is a constant: 60 minutes.
One-hour volume is the amount of fluid infused in 1 hour and is found by dividing the total volume of IV fluid by the number of hours the IV is to infuse:

$$\frac{\text{Total volume of IV fluid}}{\text{Number of hours to infuse}} = \text{One-hour volume}$$

Flow rate is the number of drops per minute (gtt/min) that the IV is to be administered.

Note: Always round your intravenous problem answers to the nearest whole number. A fraction of a drop cannot be counted.

Example

Give 1000 ml of 5% dextrose in water (D$_5$W). The IV is to run for 8 hours. The drop factor of the administration set is 10 gtt/ml.

Step 1: First divide the total volume of IV solution ordered by the number of hours the IV is to infuse to obtain the 1-hour volume:

$$\begin{array}{r} 125 \text{ ml} = 1\text{-hour volume} \\ 8 \text{ hr)}\overline{1000 \text{ ml}} = 8\text{-hour volume} \end{array}$$

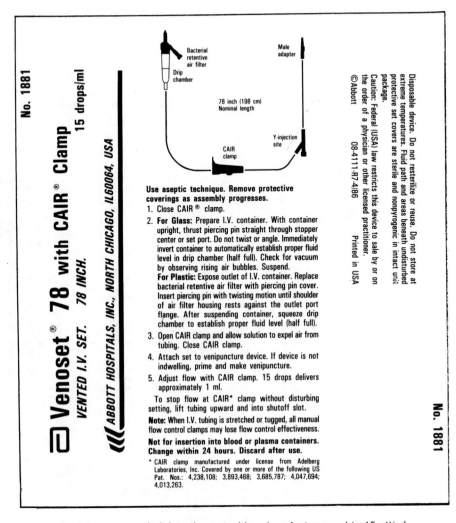

An intravenous administration set with a drop factor equal to 15 gtt/ml.

Step 2: Write the formula and substitute into it the known values:

$$\frac{\text{Drop factor}}{\text{Time}} \times \text{1-hour volume} = \text{Flow rate}$$

$$\frac{\overset{1}{\cancel{15}}\ \text{gtt/ml}}{\underset{6}{\cancel{60}}\ \text{min}} \times 125\ \text{ml} = \frac{125}{6} = 20.83 \approx 21\ \text{gtt/min}$$

Round to the nearest whole number.

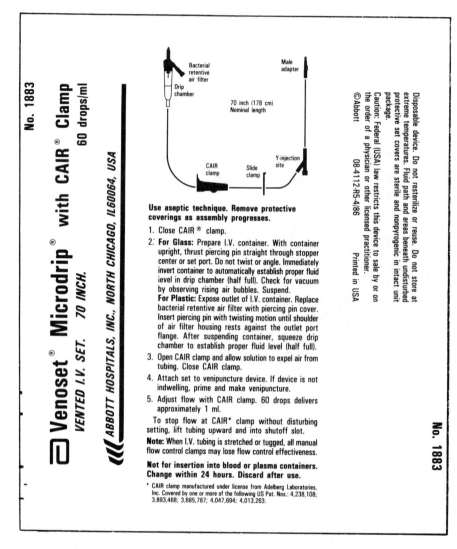

No. 1883

⊟Venoset® Microdrip® with CAIR® Clamp

60 drops/ml

VENTED I.V. SET. 70 INCH.

⟨⟨⟨ ABBOTT HOSPITALS, INC., NORTH CHICAGO, IL60064, USA

Bacterial retentive air filter

Drip chamber

Male adapter

70 inch (178 cm) Nominal length

CAIR clamp

Slide clamp

Y-injection site

Use aseptic technique. Remove protective coverings as assembly progresses.

1. Close CAIR® clamp.
2. **For Glass:** Prepare I.V. container. With container upright, thrust piercing pin straight through stopper center or set port. Do not twist or angle. Immediately invert container to automatically establish proper fluid level in drip chamber (half full). Check for vacuum by observing rising air bubbles. Suspend.
   For Plastic: Expose outlet of I.V. container. Replace bacterial retentive air filter with piercing pin cover. Insert piercing pin with twisting motion until shoulder of air filter housing rests against the outlet port flange. After suspending container, squeeze drip chamber to establish proper fluid level (half full).
3. Open CAIR clamp and allow solution to expel air from tubing. Close CAIR clamp.
4. Attach set to venipuncture device. If device is not indwelling, prime and make venipuncture.
5. Adjust flow with CAIR clamp. 60 drops delivers approximately 1 ml.

   To stop flow at CAIR* clamp without disturbing setting, lift tubing upward and into shutoff slot.

   Note: When I.V. tubing is stretched or tugged, all manual flow control clamps may lose flow control effectiveness.

   Not for insertion into blood or plasma containers. Change within 24 hours. Discard after use.

   * CAIR clamp manufactured under license from Adelberg Laboratories, Inc. Covered by one or more of the following US Pat. Nos.: 4,238,108; 3,893,468; 3,685,787; 4,047,694; 4,013,263.

No. 1883

An intravenous administration set with a drop factor equal to 60 gtt/ml.

Exercises: Large-volume IV Administration

Round your answers to the nearest whole number.

1. The doctor orders 3000 ml 5% dextrose in normal saline (D_5NS) to run for 24 hours. The drop factor of the administration set is 15 gtt/ml. At what flow rate (gtt/min) should this IV be set?

2. The doctor orders 2000 ml Ringer's lactate (RL) to run for 16 hours. The drop factor is 10 gtt/ml. At what flow rate (gtt/min) should this IV be set?

3. The doctor orders 1000 ml D_5W to run for 10 hours. The drop factor is 20 gtt/ml. At what flow rate (gtt/min) should this IV be set?

4. The doctor orders 500 ml D_5NS to run at 50 ml/hr. How many hours will this IV run? The drop factor is 60 gtt/ml. At what flow rate (gtt/min) should this IV be set?

5. The doctor orders 2500 ml D_5RL to run at 125 ml/hr. How many hours will this IV run? The drop factor is 13 gtt/ml. At what flow rate (gtt/min) should this IV be set?

Answers: Large-volume IV Administration

1.
$$3000 \text{ ml} \div 24 \text{ hr} = 125 \text{ ml/hr}$$

$$\frac{\text{Drop factor}}{\text{Time}} \times \text{1-hr volume} = \text{Flow rate}$$

$$\frac{\overset{1}{\cancel{15} \text{ gtt/ml}}}{\underset{4}{\cancel{60} \text{ min}}} \times 125 \text{ ml} = \frac{125}{4} = 31\frac{1}{4} \approx 31 \text{ gtt/min}$$

2.
$$2000 \text{ ml} \div 16 \text{ hr} = 125 \text{ ml/hr}$$

$$\frac{\overset{1}{\cancel{10}} \text{ gtt/ml}}{\underset{6}{\cancel{60}} \text{ min}} \times 125 \text{ ml} = \frac{125}{6}$$

$$= 20\frac{5}{6} \approx 21 \text{ gtt/min}$$

3.
$$1000 \text{ ml} \div 10 \text{ hr} = 100 \text{ ml/hr}$$

$$\frac{\overset{1}{\cancel{20}} \text{ gtt/ml}}{\underset{3}{\cancel{60}} \text{ min}} \times 100 \text{ ml} = \frac{100}{3}$$

$$= 33\frac{1}{3} \approx 33 \text{ gtt/min}$$

4.
$$500 \text{ ml} \div 50 \text{ ml/hr} = 10 \text{ hr (length of time the IV will run)}$$

$$\frac{\overset{1}{\cancel{60}} \text{ gtt/ml}}{\underset{1}{\cancel{60}} \text{ min}} \times 50 \text{ ml} = 50 \text{ gtt/min}$$

The 1-hour rate was ordered by the doctor.

5.
$$2500 \text{ ml} \div 125 \text{ ml/hr} = 20 \text{ hr (length of time the IV will run)}$$

$$\frac{13 \text{ gtt/ml}}{\underset{12}{\cancel{60}} \text{ min}} \times \overset{25}{\cancel{125}} \text{ ml} = \frac{325}{12}$$

$$= 27.08 \approx 27 \text{ gtt/min}$$

The 1-hour rate was ordered by the doctor.

IV CALCULATION SHORTCUT

Once you become familiar with IV flow rate calculation, you will realize that the fraction formed by placing the drop factor over 60 minutes may be reduced so that you are actually dividing the 1-hour volume by one of four numbers, depending on the IV administration set you are using. If you figure out this number for the IV set used in the hospital where you are working, you only have to divide the 1-hour volume by this "magic number" to determine the number of drops per minute at which an IV should be set to deliver the 1-hour volume.

Manufacturer	Drop Factor	Magic Number
Abbott	Approximately 15 gtt/ml	$\dfrac{15}{60} = 4$
Baxter	Approximately 10 gtt/ml	$\dfrac{10}{60} = 6$
Cutter	Approximately 20 gtt/ml	$\dfrac{20}{60} = 3$
Any mini or micro dropper	Approximately 60 gtt/ml	$\dfrac{60}{60} = 1$

Example

The physician orders an IV to be run at 125 ml/hr. Calculate the flow rate (gtt/min) for each of the administration sets.

$$\frac{\text{Drop factor}}{60 \text{ min}} \times 1\text{-hr volume} = \text{Flow rate}$$

If we use a set that flows 15 gtt/ml

$$\frac{\overset{1}{\cancel{15}}}{\underset{4}{\cancel{60}}} \times 125 = \frac{125}{\textcircled{4}} = 31\frac{1}{4} \approx 31 \text{ gtt/min}$$

If we use a set that flows 10 gtt/ml

$$\frac{\overset{1}{\cancel{10}}}{\underset{6}{\cancel{60}}} \times 125 = \frac{125}{\textcircled{6}} = 20\frac{5}{6} \approx 21 \text{ gtt/min}$$

If we use a set that flows 20 gtt/ml

$$\frac{\overset{1}{\cancel{20}}}{\underset{3}{\cancel{60}}} \times 125 = \frac{125}{\textcircled{3}} = 41\frac{2}{3} \approx 42 \text{ gtt/min}$$

If we use a micro set that flows 60 gtt/ml

$$\frac{\overset{1}{\cancel{60}}}{\underset{1}{\cancel{60}}} \times 125 = \frac{125}{\textcircled{1}} = 125 \text{ gtt/min}$$

Note: In each case above, the magic number is circled. Some IV sets used for administering special solutions may have a different flow rate. Use the formula to calculate the flow rate as above. Always be sure to check for the drop factor and regulate the IV accordingly.

Many hospitals use infusion pumps or controllers to administer IV infusions. These machines deliver the IV fluid at a rate preset on the machine. So you may ask, "Why do I need to know how to calculate the IV formula?" The fact is that few hospitals have all of the infusion equipment needed. Therefore, you must know the formula to calculate IV infusion rates when volume control machines are not available.

SMALL-VOLUME IV ADMINISTRATION

Medications are frequently administered to patients in 50 to 100 ml of IV fluid. The administration time may be 30 to 60 minutes. The length of time for administration and the dilution of the drug depends on the stability or the irritability, or both, of the particular drug. See drug guidelines or consult the pharmacist. The IV should be maintained at the correct flow rate to prevent complications.

To calculate the flow rate of small-volume IVs use the same formula as was used to calculate the large volume IV flow rate, substituting the actual time of administration and the volume to be administered:

Formula:

$$\frac{\text{Drop factor}}{\text{Time}} \times \text{Volume} = \text{Flow rate}$$

In small volume IVs the **drop factor** and the **flow rate** are the same as for large volume IVs.

The **time** is usually less than 1 hour (i.e., 15, 20, 45 minutes).

Volume refers to the total volume to be infused (rather than, as with large-volume IVs, the volume to be infused within 1 hour).

Example

Administer 0.5 g of Kefzol in 100 ml of IV solution over 45 minutes (see label). The drop factor is 20 gtt/ml. At what flow rate (gtt/min) must this IV run?

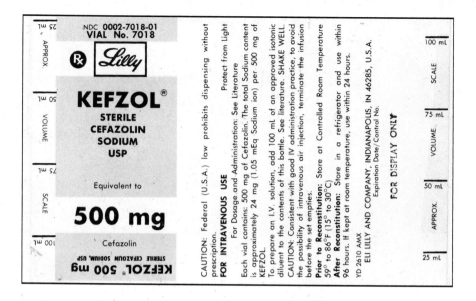

$$\frac{\text{Drop factor}}{\text{Time}} \times \text{Volume} = \text{Flow rate (gtt/min)}$$

$$\frac{\overset{4}{\cancel{20}} \text{ gtt/ml}}{\underset{9}{\cancel{45}} \text{ min}} \times 100 \text{ ml} = \frac{400}{9} = 44.4 \approx 44 \text{ gtt/min}$$

Exercises: Small-volume IV Administration

Round your answers to the nearest whole number.

1. You are to administer 300 mg kanamycin in 100 ml IV fluid over 30 minutes. The drop factor is 15 gtt/ml. What flow rate (gtt/min) should you use?

2. The physician's order calls for 100 mg gentamicin in 150 ml IV fluid over 60 minutes. The drop factor is 10 gtt/ml. What flow rate should be used?

3. You are to administer 170 mg tobramycin in 125 ml IV fluid over 45 minutes. The drop factor is 20 gtt/ml. At how many drops per minute should the IV be set?

4. The physician's order calls for 3 g mezlocillin sodium q4h (every 4 hours) in 100 ml solution over 40 minutes. The drop factor is 60 gtt/ml. What flow rate should you use?

5. You are to administer 4 g $MgSO_4$ in 250 ml D_5W over 20 minutes, stat (at once). The drop factor is 60 gtt/ml. At what flow rate should the IV be set?

Answers: Small-volume IV Administration

$$\frac{\text{Drop factor}}{\text{Time}} \times \text{Volume} = \text{Flow rate (gtt/min)}$$

1.
$$\frac{\overset{1}{\cancel{15}} \text{ gtt/ml}}{\underset{2}{\cancel{30}} \text{ min}} \times 100 \text{ ml} = \frac{100}{2}$$
$$= 50 \text{ gtt/min kanamycin solution}$$

2.
$$\frac{\overset{1}{\cancel{10}} \text{ gtt/ml}}{\underset{6}{\cancel{60}} \text{ min}} \times 150 \text{ ml} = \frac{150}{6}$$
$$= 25 \text{ gtt/min gentamicin solution}$$

3.
$$\frac{\overset{4}{\cancel{20}} \text{ gtt/ml}}{\underset{9}{\cancel{45}} \text{ min}} \times 125 \text{ ml} = \frac{500}{9}$$
$$= 55.56 \approx 56 \text{ gtt/min tobramycin solution}$$

4.
$$\frac{\overset{3}{\cancel{60}} \text{ gtt/ml}}{\underset{\underset{1}{2}}{\cancel{40}} \text{ min}} \times \overset{50}{\cancel{100}} \text{ ml} = 150 \text{ gtt/min mezlocillin solution}$$

5.

$$\frac{\overset{3}{\cancel{60} \text{ gtt/ml}}}{\underset{1}{\cancel{20} \text{ min}}} \times 250 \text{ ml} = 750 \text{ gtt/min magnesium sulfate solution}$$

This IV is flowing rather than dropping. You could not count 750 gtt/min.

VOLUME CONTROL SETS

A volume control set is used to administer IV fluids or IV medications to infants or young children. It is also used to control the fluid volume for older children and adults, especially when there is circulatory, heart, or kidney involvement. The Buretrol (see picture on page 140), Soluset, Pediatrol, and Volutrol are examples of these sets. The volume control set is an IV line with a fluid chamber that will hold 100 to 150 ml of fluid. For accurate fluid measurement, the chamber is calibrated at 2-ml intervals. These sets employ a microdrip (60 gtt/ml) delivery system. They are used to prevent infusion of a larger volume of fluid than the patient could tolerate. Today, volume control pumps and controllers have reduced the usage of these volume control sets in the hospital, although they may be used along with a pump to administer IV medications. They are, however, being used increasingly to administer IV medication to patients in the home.

When using the volume control set, you fill the chamber with enough fluid to infuse for a specified amount of time.

Example 1

Infuse the IV at a rate of 30 ml/hr. If only IV fluid is being infused, the IV control chamber may be filled with a 1- or 2-hour volume of fluid.

The drip rate is set according to the volume being infused per hour, in this example, 30 ml. The drop factor is 60 gtt/ml, therefore, the drop rate will be 30 gtt/min:

$$\frac{\overset{1}{\cancel{60} \text{ gtt/ml}}}{\underset{1}{\cancel{60} \text{ min}}} \times 30 \text{ ml} = 30 \text{ gtt/min}$$

If medication is to be infused, only the amount of fluid to administer the medication in the specified time period is put in the IV control chamber. Neither the hourly volume nor drop rate should be changed. If possible, give the medication within a fraction of the total hourly volume.

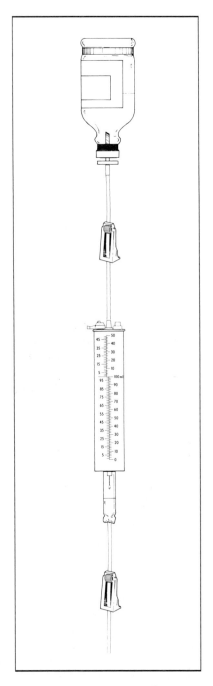

Buretrol volume control set.

Example 2

The physician orders 10 mg of gentamicin IV q8h via Buretrol over 30 minutes. The infant is already receiving 30 ml/hr of IV fluids. The drop factor is 60 gtt/ml. You have gentamicin 10 mg/ml.

Questions
How much gentamicin solution must be added to the Buretrol?
How much additional IV fluid must be added?
What is the drop rate for this IV?

Answers
The strength of the gentamicin is 10 mg/ml so you need to add 1 ml of gentamicin to the Buretrol. Since the IV is running at 30 ml/hr and the medicine is to be given in 30 minutes, one half or 15 ml of solution is needed in the Buretrol. You need to add to the 1 ml of gentamicin 14 ml of IV fluid to administer the drug in 30 minutes.

Note: It may be necessary to solve a dosage problem to determine the amount of medication to add to the IV control chamber.

Exercises: Volume Control Sets

1. The physician's order calls for 20 mg gentamicin IV over a 2-hour period using a Soluset. The child is receiving fluid at the rate of 40 ml/hr. The drop factor is 60 gtt/ml. The gentamicin is available as 60 mg per 1.5 ml.

   a. How many milliliters of gentamicin will you add?

   b. How much fluid?

   c. What flow rate will you use?

2. The physician's order calls for tobramycin 60 mg IV via a Buretrol over 45 minutes. The child is receiving 60 ml/hr of IV fluid. The tobramycin is available as 80 mg per 2 ml. The drop factor is 60 gtt/ml.

   a. How many milliliters of tobramycin will you add?

   b. How much fluid?

   c. What flow rate will you use?

3. You need to administer 500 mg kanamycin in 40 minutes. The patient's IV is infusing at 150 ml/hr via a Buretrol. You have a vial that contains 1 g of kanamycin per 3 ml of solution. The drop factor is 60 gtt/ml.

   a. How many milliliters of kanamycin will you add to the Buretrol?

   b. How much fluid?

   c. What flow rate will you use?

4. You need to administer 1 g Gantrisin q6h for 30 minutes. You have ampules of Gantrisin containing 2 g per 5 ml. The patient is receiving fluid at the rate of 70 ml/hr via a Soluset. The drop factor is 60 gtt/ml.

   a. How many milliliters of Gantrisin will you add?

   b. How much fluid?

   c. What flow rate will you use?

5. The order calls for 300 mg clindamycin (Cleocin) IV over 20 minutes. The patient is receiving IV fluid at the rate of 150 ml/hr via a Soluset. You have 4-ml ampules containing 600 mg Cleocin. The drop factor is 60 gtt/ml.

   a. How many milliliters of Cleocin will you add?

   b. How many ml of IV fluid?

   c. What flow rate will you use?

Answers: Volume Control Sets

1. a.
$$\frac{1}{\cancel{20}\text{ mg}} \times 1.5 \text{ ml} = \frac{1.5}{3} = 0.5 \text{ ml}$$

$$\frac{60 \text{ mg}}{1.5 \text{ ml}} :: \frac{20 \text{ mg}}{x \text{ ml}}$$
$$60x = 30$$
$$x = 0.5 \text{ ml}$$

Add 0.5 ml gentamicin to the IV.

b. Since the gentamicin is to run over 2 hours, and the volume to be infused is 40 ml/hr, a total of 80 ml is required. You therefore need to add 0.5 ml of gentamicin and 79.5 ml IV fluid to the Soluset.

c. Infuse at

$$\frac{\overset{1}{\cancel{60} \text{ gtt/ml}}}{\underset{1}{\cancel{60} \text{ min}}} \times 40 \text{ ml} = 40 \text{ gtt/min}$$

OR

$$\frac{\overset{1}{\cancel{60} \text{ gtt/ml}}}{\underset{1}{\underset{2}{\cancel{120} \text{ min}}}} \times \overset{40}{\cancel{80}} \text{ ml} = 40 \text{ gtt/min}$$

2. a.

$$\frac{\overset{3}{\cancel{60} \text{ mg}}}{\underset{4}{\cancel{80} \text{ mg}}} \times 2 \text{ ml} = \frac{6}{4}$$

$$= 1.5 \text{ ml}$$

$$\frac{80 \text{ mg}}{2 \text{ ml}} :: \frac{60 \text{ mg}}{x \text{ ml}}$$
$$80x = 120$$
$$x = 1.5 \text{ ml}$$

Add 1.5 ml of tobramycin to the Buretrol.

b. Since the IV is to run over 45 minutes, and the infusion rate of the Buretrol is 60 ml/hr, we can determine the number of milliliters of IV fluid to be infused in 45 minutes by solving the following ratio:

$$\frac{60 \text{ ml}}{60 \text{ min}} :: \frac{x \text{ ml}}{45 \text{ min}}$$
$$60x = 2700$$
$$x = 45 \text{ ml}$$

Because a total of 45 ml of fluid must be added to the Buretrol, and you need to add 1.5 ml tobramycin, you must add 43.5 ml IV fluid as well.

c. Infuse at

$$\frac{60 \text{ gtt/ml}}{45 \text{ min}} \times 45 \text{ ml} = 60 \text{ gtt/min}$$

3. a.

$$\frac{\overset{1}{\cancel{500} \text{ mg}}}{\underset{2}{\cancel{1000} \text{ mg}}} \times 3 \text{ ml} = \frac{3}{2}$$

$$= 1.5 \text{ ml}$$

$$\frac{1000 \text{ mg}}{3 \text{ ml}} :: \frac{500 \text{ mg}}{x \text{ ml}}$$
$$1000x = 1500$$
$$x = 1.5 \text{ ml}$$

Add 1.5 ml kanamycin to the Buretrol.

b. A total of 100 ml must be added to the Buretrol:

100 ml total fluid

$-\underline{1.5\ ml}$ kanamycin

98.5 ml of IV fluid

$$\frac{150\ ml}{60\ min} :: \frac{x\ ml}{40\ min}$$

$$60x = 6000$$

$$x = 100\ ml/40\ min$$

Therefore add 98.5 ml IV fluid to the Buretrol.

c. Infuse at

$$\frac{\cancel{60}\ gtt/ml}{\cancel{40}\ min} \times 100\ ml = 150\ gtt/min$$

4. a. $$\frac{1\ g}{2\ g} \times 5\ ml = \frac{5}{2}$$

$$= 2.5\ ml$$

$$\frac{2\ g}{5\ ml} :: \frac{1\ g}{x\ ml}$$

$$2x = 5$$

$$x = 2.5\ ml$$

Add 2.5 ml Gantrisin to the Soluset.

b. A total of 35 ml must be added to the Soluset:

35 ml total fluid

$-\underline{2.5\ ml}$ Gantrisin

32.5 ml of IV fluid

$$\frac{70\ ml}{60\ min} = \frac{x\ ml}{30\ min}$$

$$60\ x = 2100$$

$$x = 35\ ml/30\ min$$

Therefore add 32.5 ml IV fluid to the Soluset.

c. Infuse at

$$\frac{\overset{2}{\cancel{60}}\ gtt/ml}{\underset{1}{\cancel{30}}\ min} \times 35\ ml = 70\ gtt/min$$

5. a. $$\frac{\overset{1}{\cancel{300}\ mg}}{\underset{2}{\cancel{600}\ mg}} \times 4\ ml = \frac{4}{2}$$

$$= 2\ ml$$

$$\frac{600\ mg}{4\ ml} :: \frac{300\ mg}{x\ ml}$$

$$600x = 1200$$

$$x = 2\ ml$$

Add 2 ml Cleocin to the Soluset.

b. A total of 50 ml must be added to the Soluset:

50 ml total fluid
− 2 ml Cleosin
48 ml of IV fluid

$$\frac{150 \text{ ml}}{60 \text{ min}} = \frac{x \text{ ml}}{20 \text{ min}}$$

$$60\, x = 3000$$

$$x = 50 \text{ ml/20 min}$$

Therefore add 48 ml of IV fluid to the Soluset.

c. Infuse at

$$\frac{\overset{3}{\cancel{60} \text{ gtt/ml}}}{\underset{1}{\cancel{20} \text{ min}}} \times 50 \text{ ml} = 150 \text{ gtt/min}$$

LARGE-VOLUME IVs CONTAINING IV DRUGS

Drugs may be ordered around the clock or to run for several hours in a large volume IV (500 to 1000 ml). The doctor will order the IV to run at a certain number of g, mEq, or units per hour. Think of this problem as a dosage problem. The only difference is the volume of fluid involved.

Example

The doctor orders 1000 ml D_5W with 20 mEq KCl added, to be administered at the rate of 2 mEq/hr. (Dose ordered: 2 mEq/hour. Strength on hand: 20 mEq/1000 ml.)

Method 1:

$$\frac{\text{The dose ordered}}{\text{Strength on hand}} \times \text{vehicle} = \text{Amount to give}$$

$$\frac{2 \text{ mEq}}{\underset{1}{\cancel{20} \text{ mEq}}} \times \overset{50}{\cancel{1000}} \text{ ml} = 100 \text{ ml to be administered per hour}$$

Method 2:

Drug : Vehicle : : Drug desired : Amount of vehicle to administer

20 mEq : 1000 ml : : 2 mEq : x ml

$$20x = 2000$$

$$x = 100 \text{ ml to be administered per hour}$$

Once the volume of drug to be administered is determined, set up an

IV problem using the drop factor of the IV administration set you are to use and determine the drops per minute to run the IV.

Exercises: Large-volume IVs Containing Drugs

1. Physician's order: Add 10 g $MgSO_4$ to 1000 ml D_5W. Run at 1 g $MgSO_4$ per hour. How much fluid will be needed to administer 1 g $MgSO_4$ per hour? If the drop factor for the IV set is 60 gtt/ml, at how many drops per minute should this IV be set?

2. The patient in Exercise 1 improves. The physician reduces the dose to 500 mg $MgSO_4$ per hour. How much fluid will be needed to administer this dosage? If the drop factor is 60 gtt/ml, what flow rate (gtt/min) should be used?

3. Physician's order: Add 200 U Regular insulin in 500 ml $D_5\frac{1}{2}NS$ and run at 25 U/hr. How much fluid should infuse per hour? What flow rate (gtt/min) should be used if the drop factor is 20 gtt/ml?

4. Physician's order: Add 1000 mcg Levophed to 500 ml of IV solution. Run at 180 mcg/hr. How much fluid should infuse per hour? The drop factor is 15 gtt/ml. What flow rate (gtt/min) should be used?

5. Physician's order: Administer 120 mg lidocaine per hour. Add 480 mg to 500 ml of solution. How much solution is needed to administer 120 mg/hr? If the drop factor is 10 gtt/ml, at how many drops per minute should the IV be set?

Answers: Large-volume IVs Containing Drugs

1. $$\frac{1 \text{ g/hr}}{\cancel{10} \text{ g}} \times \cancel{1000}^{\,100} \text{ ml} = 100 \text{ ml/hr}$$
    $$\underset{1}{}$$

    $$10 \text{ g} : 1000 \text{ ml} :: 1 \text{ g/hr} : x \text{ ml}$$
    $$\frac{10 \text{ g}}{1000 \text{ ml}} :: \frac{1 \text{ g/hr}}{x \text{ ml}}$$
    $$10x = 1000$$
    $$x = 100 \text{ ml/hr}$$

    $$\frac{60 \text{ gtt/ml}}{60 \text{ min}} \times 100 \text{ ml} = 100 \text{ gtt/min needed to administer}$$
    $$1 \text{ g of } MgSO_4 \text{ per hour}$$

2. $$500 \text{ mg} = 0.5 \text{ g}$$
    $$\frac{0.5 \text{ g/hr}}{\cancel{10} \text{ gm}} \times \cancel{1000}^{\,100} \text{ ml} = 50.0 \text{ ml/hr}$$
    $$\underset{1}{}$$

    $$10 \text{ g} : 1000 \text{ ml} :: 0.5 \text{ g/hr} : x \text{ ml}$$
    $$\frac{10 \text{ g}}{1000 \text{ ml}} :: \frac{0.5 \text{ g/hr}}{x \text{ ml}}$$
    $$10x = 500$$
    $$x = 50 \text{ ml/hr}$$

    $$\frac{60 \text{ gtt/ml}}{60 \text{ min}} \times 50 \text{ ml} = 50 \text{ gtt/min}$$

3. $$\frac{25 \text{ U/hr}}{\underset{2}{\cancel{200} \text{ U}}} \times \cancel{500}^{\,5} \text{ ml} = \frac{125}{2}$$
    $$= 62.5 \text{ ml/hr}$$

    $$200 \text{ U} : 500 \text{ ml} :: 25 \text{ U/hr} : x \text{ ml}$$
    $$\frac{200 \text{ U}}{500 \text{ ml}} :: \frac{25 \text{ U/hr}}{x \text{ ml}}$$
    $$200x = 12,500$$
    $$x = 62.5 \text{ ml/hr}$$

    $$\frac{\overset{1}{\cancel{20} \text{ gtt/ml}}}{\underset{3}{\cancel{60} \text{ min}}} \times 62.5 \text{ ml} = \frac{62.5}{3} = 20.8 \approx 21 \text{ gtt/min}$$

4. $$\frac{\overset{90}{180 \text{ mcg/hr}}}{\underset{1}{\underset{500}{1000 \text{ mcg}}}} \times \cancel{500}^{\,1} \text{ ml} = 90 \text{ ml/hr}$$

    $$1000 \text{ mcg} : 500 \text{ ml} :: 180 \text{ mcg/hr} : x \text{ ml}$$
    $$\frac{1000 \text{ mcg}}{500 \text{ ml}} :: \frac{180 \text{ mcg/hr}}{x \text{ ml}}$$
    $$1,000x = 90,000$$
    $$x = 90 \text{ ml/hr}$$

    $$\frac{\overset{1}{\cancel{15} \text{ gtt/ml}}}{\underset{4}{\cancel{60} \text{ min}}} \times 90 \text{ ml} = \frac{90}{4} = 22.5 \approx 23 \text{ gtt/min}$$

5.   1

$$\frac{\overset{1}{\cancel{120}}\text{ mg/hr}}{\underset{4}{\cancel{480}}\text{ mg}} \times 500 \text{ ml} = \frac{500}{4}$$

$$= 125 \text{ ml/hr}$$

$$480 \text{ mg} : 500 \text{ ml} :: 120 \text{ mg/hr} : x \text{ ml}$$

$$\frac{480 \text{ mg}}{500 \text{ ml}} :: \frac{120 \text{ mg/hr}}{x \text{ ml}}$$

$$480x = 60,000$$

$$x = 125 \text{ ml/hr}$$

$$\frac{\overset{1}{\cancel{10}}\text{ gtt/ml}}{\underset{6}{\cancel{60}}\text{ min}} \times 125 \text{ ml} = \frac{125}{6} = 20.8 \approx 21 \text{ gtt/min}$$

Each of these medications would probably be administered using an IV controller or pump. You would use the 1-hour volume to set the rate control

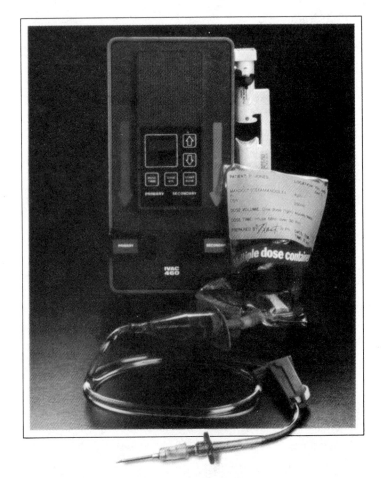

IV infusion pump showing IV bag containing the drug Mandol.

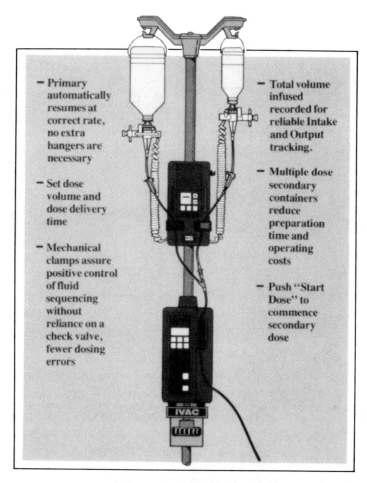

A single IV pump that delivers both a primary and secondary IV infusion.

on the machine, and set the machine for the specific drops per minute found on the machine. Meanwhile, you have obtained more experience with IV rate calculations.

IV MEDICATION ADMINISTERED PER MINUTE

The physician may order the IV rate for a drug to infuse per minute instead of per hour. You can determine the amount of drug to infuse per minute by using the dosage formula or ratio and proportion.

To determine the IV flow rate, use the small volume IV fluid formula:

$$\frac{\text{Drop factor}}{\text{Time}} \times \text{Volume} = \text{Flow rate}$$

Example

Administer procainamide at 3 mg/min. You have 500 ml IV fluid with 1 g of procainamide. How many milliliters per minute should this IV infuse? If the drop factor is 60 gtt/ml, how many drops per minute should the IV infuse?

Step 1: You need to solve a dosage problem to find out how much fluid to infuse per minute.

<table>
<tr><td align="center">**Formula**</td><td align="center">**Ratio**</td></tr>
<tr><td>$\dfrac{3 \text{ mg/min}}{1000 \text{ mg}} \times 500 \text{ ml} = \dfrac{3}{2}$</td><td>$\dfrac{1000 \text{ mg}}{500 \text{ ml}} :: \dfrac{3 \text{ mg/min}}{x \text{ ml}}$</td></tr>
<tr><td align="center">$= 1.5 \text{ ml/min}$</td><td align="center">$1000x = 1500$</td></tr>
<tr><td></td><td align="center">$x = 1.5 \text{ ml/min}$</td></tr>
</table>

Run the IV at 1.5 ml/min.

Step 2:   **IV Formula**

$$\frac{\text{Drop factor}}{\text{Time}} \times \text{Volume} = \text{Flow rate}$$

$$\frac{60 \text{ gtt/ml}}{1 \text{ min}} \times 1.5 \text{ ml} = 90 \text{ gtt/min}$$

Since the time is 1 minute, you can simply multiply the 1-minute volume by the drop factor:

$$\text{Drop factor} \times \text{1-minute volume} = \text{Drops per minute}$$
$$60 \text{ gtt/ml} \times 1.5 \text{ ml/min} = 90 \text{ gtt/min}$$

Exercises: IV Medication Administered per Minute

1. Physician's order: Add 2 g of Xylocaine to 500 ml D$_5$W. Run at 2 mg/min. How many milliliters of fluid will you give per minute? If the drop factor is 60 gtt/ml, at how many drops per minute should the IV be set?

2. Physician's order: Add 1000 mcg of Levophed to 500 ml IV solution. Run at 3 mcg/min. How many milliliters of fluid will you give per minute? At how many drops per minute should the IV be set if the drop factor is 20 gtt/ml? If the drop factor is 60 gtt/ml?

3. Physician's order: For a 3-kg infant, add 45 mg of dopamine to 100 ml D$_5$W. Run at 15 mcg/min. How many milliliters of fluid will you give per minute to administer 15 mcg of dopamine? At how many drops per minute should the IV be set if the drop factor is 60 gtt/ml?

4. Physician's order: Administer lidocaine 0.03 mg/kg/min by IV infusion to an infant weighing 4.6 kg. The drop factor is 60 gtt/ml. You have lidocaine 66 mg per 32 ml. How many milliliters of fluid will you give per minute? At what flow rate (gtt/min) should the IV be set?

5. Physician's order: Administer lidocaine 40 mcg/min. You have a 0.2% solution (2 g of lidocaine per 1000 ml). The drop factor is 60 gtt/ml. How many milliliters of fluid will you give per minute? At what flow rate (gtt/min) should this IV be set?

Answers: IV Medication Administered per Minute

1. 2 mg = 0.002 g

$$\frac{\overset{0.001}{\cancel{0.002}}\text{ g/min}}{\underset{1}{\cancel{2}\text{ g}}} \times 500 \text{ ml} = 0.5 \text{ ml/min}$$

$$\frac{2 \text{ g}}{500 \text{ ml}} :: \frac{0.002 \text{ g/min}}{x \text{ ml/min}}$$
$$2x = 1$$
$$x = 0.5 \text{ ml/min}$$

Administer Xylocaine at the rate of 0.5 ml/min. Infuse at

$$0.5 \text{ ml} \times 60 \text{ gtt/ml} = 30 \text{ gtt/min}$$

2.

$$\frac{3 \text{ mcg/min}}{\underset{2}{\cancel{1000}}\text{ mcg}} \times \overset{1}{\cancel{500}} \text{ ml} = \frac{3}{2}$$
$$= 1.5 \text{ ml/min}$$

$$\frac{1000 \text{ mcg}}{500 \text{ ml}} :: \frac{3 \text{ mcg/min}}{x \text{ ml/min}}$$
$$1000x = 1500$$
$$x = 1.5 \text{ ml/min}$$

Administer Levophed at the rate of 1.5 ml/min. Infuse at

$$1.5 \text{ ml/min} \times 20 \text{ gtt/ml} = 30 \text{ gtt/min}$$

$$1.5 \text{ ml/min} \times 60 \text{ gtt/ml} = 90 \text{ gtt/min}$$

3. 45 mg = 45,000 mcg

$$\dfrac{15 \text{ mcg/min}}{\underset{450}{\cancel{45,000} \text{ mcg}}} \times \overset{1}{\cancel{100}} \text{ ml} = \dfrac{15}{450}$$

$$\dfrac{45,000 \text{ mcg}}{100 \text{ ml}} :: \dfrac{15 \text{ mcg/min}}{x \text{ ml/min}}$$

$$45,000x = 1500$$

$$= 0.033 \text{ ml/min} \qquad x = 0.033 \text{ ml/min}$$

Administer dopamine at the rate of 0.033 ml/min. Infuse at

$$0.033 \text{ ml/min} \times 60 \text{ gtt/ml} = 1.98 \approx 2 \text{ gtt/min}$$

4. 0.03 mg/kg/min × 4.6 kg = 0.138 mg/min of lidocaine

$$\dfrac{0.138 \text{ mg/min}}{66 \text{ mg}} \times 32 \text{ ml} = \dfrac{4.416}{66}$$

$$\dfrac{66 \text{ mg}}{32 \text{ ml}} :: \dfrac{0.138 \text{ mg/min}}{x \text{ ml/min}}$$

$$66x = 4.416$$

$$= 0.066 \text{ ml/min} \qquad x = 0.066 \text{ ml/min}$$

Administer 0.066 ml lidocaine solution per minute. Infuse at

$$60 \text{ gtt/ml} \times 0.066 = 3.96 \approx 4 \text{ gtt/min}$$

5.
$$2 \text{ g} = 2000 \text{ mg}$$
$$40 \text{ mcg} = 0.040 \text{ mg}$$

$$\dfrac{0.04 \text{ mg/min}}{\underset{2}{\cancel{2000} \text{ mg}}} \times \overset{1}{\cancel{1000}} \text{ ml} = 0.02 \text{ ml/min}$$

$$\dfrac{2000 \text{ mg}}{1000 \text{ ml}} :: \dfrac{0.040 \text{ mg/min}}{x \text{ ml/min}}$$

$$2000x = 40$$

$$x = 0.02 \text{ ml/min}$$

Administer 0.02 ml of lidocaine per minute. Infuse at

$$0.02 \text{ ml/min} \times 60 \text{ gtt/ml} = 1.2 \text{ gtt/min}$$

Note: To administer lidocaine hydrochloride, or any potent medication, by continuous intravenous infusion you should use a precision volume control IV set.*

IVs RUNNING OFF SCHEDULE

More often than we care to admit, IV infusions run off schedule if volume control machines are not used. The patient may move his or her arm and either speed up or slow down the rate of flow. The tubing may be kinked or the patient may be lying on the tubing. The person responsible for mon-

* *Physician's Desk Reference,* RN edition, 1981, p. 532.

itoring the IV must correct the situation by the following steps:

1. Determine the volume to be infused per hour and the drop factor.
2. Determine how much fluid should have infused.
3. Determine how much fluid is in the IV bottle (bag).
4. Recalculate the IV rate using the new volume and the hours remaining to infuse if the IV is not on time.
5. *Do not* try to catch up an IV by running it fast until the IV is caught up. This practice could have very serious consequences, especially with infants or young children, geriatric patients, or any patient with renal, heart, or circulatory impairment.
6. Spread the extra fluid volume over the remaining time. By spreading the volume out over a longer period of time, only a small increase in volume is necessary.

Example 1

At 8:00 AM, a 1000-ml bag of D$_5$RL is hung. The flow rate is 125 ml/hr and the drop factor is 20 gtt/ml. At 12:00 noon there is 550 ml left. Is this IV on time?

In 4 hours, 500 ml should have infused:

$$4 \text{ hr} \times 125 \text{ ml/hr} = 500 \text{ ml}$$

If 550 ml remains, 350 ml has already infused. Therefore, the IV is 50 ml behind schedule.

The IV has 4 more hours to infuse. You recalculate the infusion rate by dividing the remaining volume by the remaining hours of infusion:

$$137.5 \text{ ml/hr} = \text{New 1 hr vol}$$
$$4 \text{ hr})\overline{550.0} \text{ ml} = \text{Volume remaining}$$

It will be necessary to speed up the IV by only 12.5 ml/hr to infuse the 1000 ml of fluid in 8 hours as ordered:

$$137.5 \text{ ml/hr new rate}$$
$$- 125 \text{ ml/hr original rate}$$
$$\overline{12.5} \text{ ml/hr increase in rate}$$

You can recalculate the IV flow rate by substituting the new volume into the IV flow rate formula:

$$\frac{\text{Drop factor}}{\text{Time}} \times \text{volume} = \text{Flow rate}$$

$$\frac{20 \text{ gtt/ml}}{60 \text{ min}} \times 137.5 \text{ ml} = 45.8 \approx 46 \text{ gtt/min}$$

The original flow rate was 42 gtt/min. The new rate is only 4 gtt/min more.

Example 2

At 3:00 PM you have 500 ml IV fluid left in the bottle. The rate is 50 ml/hr and the drop factor is 15 gtt/ml. At 8:00 PM you have 200 ml left. Is this IV on time?

$$\frac{10 \text{ hr}}{50 \overline{)500} \text{ ml}}$$

At 50 cc/hr there was enough fluid in the bottle to last 10 hours; in 5 hours 250 ml should have been infused. However, 200 ml remain. 300 ml has been infused. The IV is 50 ml ahead of schedule.

You recalculate the infusion rate as follows:

$$\frac{40 \text{ ml/hr}}{5 \overline{)200} \text{ total volume left}}$$

The flow rate is determined by substituting the new 1 hr volume:

$$\frac{\overset{1}{\cancel{15}} \text{ gtt/ml}}{\underset{\underset{1}{\cancel{4}}}{\cancel{60} \text{ min}}} \times \overset{10}{\cancel{40}} \text{ ml} = 10 \text{ gtt/min}$$

Exercises: IVs Running Off Schedule

1. At 9:00 AM 500 ml D₅W is started and set to infuse at 20 ml/hr. The drop factor is 60 gtt/ml. At 3:00 PM how much fluid should be left? If there is 425 ml left, what is your next step? (Calculate correction.)

2. When you arrived for the night shift at 11:00 PM the evening nurse reported that Mrs. Knight's IV was running on time. There was 625 ml remaining in the 1-L IV bag. The IV is to be infused at 125 ml/hr. At 1:00 AM you discover that there is 450 ml left. Is the IV on time? The drop factor is 10 gtt/ml. Calculate any correction necessary.

3. At 12:00 noon, a 1000-ml IV of D_5RL is hung. It is to run at 100 ml/hr. The drop factor is 15 gtt/ml. At 6:00 PM there is 500 ml left. Is this IV on time? Calculate any corrections.

Answers: IVs Running Off Schedule

1. Since 9:00 AM, 6 hours has elapsed. At 20 ml/hr, 120 ml of fluid should have infused:

$$20 \text{ ml/hr} \times 6 \text{ hr} = 120 \text{ ml}$$

If the IV is on time, 380 ml should be left in the bottle $(500 - 120 = 380$ ml). The 500-ml bottle running at 20 ml/hr would run for 25 hours:

$$\begin{array}{r} 25 \text{ hours} \\ 20 \text{ ml}\overline{)500} \end{array}$$

Since 6 hours have elapsed, 19 hours remain. Recalculate the IV infusion rate as follows:

$$\begin{array}{r} 22.36 \approx 22 \text{ ml/hr} \\ 19\overline{)425.00} \\ \underline{38} \\ 45 \\ \underline{38} \\ 70 \\ \underline{57} \\ 130 \\ \underline{114} \\ 11 \end{array}$$

Infuse at

$$\frac{\overset{1}{\cancel{60} \text{ gtt/ml}}}{\underset{1}{\cancel{60} \text{ min}}} \times 22 \text{ ml} = 22 \text{ gtt/min}$$

2.   625 ml in bag at 11:00 PM.

   $\underline{-\ 250}$ ml should have infused by 1:00 AM

   375 ml should be left

The IV is 75 ml behind schedule.

$$\frac{3 \text{ hr time remaining}}{125)\overline{375} \text{ ml}}$$
$$\frac{375}{0}$$

$$\frac{150 \text{ ml/hr}}{3)\overline{450} \text{ ml}}$$
$$\frac{3}{15}$$
$$\underline{15}$$

Run the IV at 150 ml/hr. Infuse at

$$\frac{\overset{1}{\cancel{10}} \text{ gtt/ml}}{\underset{6}{\cancel{60}} \text{ min}} \times 150 \text{ ml} = \frac{150}{6} = 25 \text{ gtt/min}$$

3. At a rate of 100 ml/hr, 600 ml should have infused in 6 hours, leaving 400 ml. However, 500 ml remain, so the IV is 100 ml behind:

$$\begin{array}{r} 600 \text{ ml} \\ - 500 \text{ ml} \\ \hline 100 \text{ ml behind} \end{array}$$

Recalculate the infusion rate:

$$\frac{125}{4)\overline{500}} = \frac{\text{1 hour volume}}{\text{= volume left}}$$

Infuse at

$$\frac{\overset{1}{\cancel{15}} \text{ gtt/ml}}{\underset{4}{\cancel{60}} \text{ min}} \times 125 \text{ ml} = \frac{125}{4}$$

$$= 31.25 \approx 31 \text{ gtt/min}$$

PROBLEMS: INTRAVENOUS FLUID RATE CALCULATION

1. The physician orders 3000 ml IV fluid to run for 24 hours. The administration set drop factor is 10 gtt/ml. At what flow rate (gtt/min) must the nurse run this IV?

2. The physician orders 1500 ml IV fluid to run for 10 hours. The administration set drop factor is 20 gtt/ml. At what flow rate (gtt/min) must the nurse run this IV?

3. The physician orders 240 ml IV fluid for an infant, to run for 24 hours. The IV administration set drop factor is 60 gtt/ml. How fast must the nurse run this IV?

4. The physician orders 2500 ml IV fluid to infuse for 24 hours. The IV administration set drop factor is 15 gtt/ml. At what flow rate (gtt/min) must this IV be set?

5. The physician orders 3000 ml IV fluid to be infused in 16 hours. The IV administration drop factor is 10 gtt/ml. How fast must the nurse run this IV?

6. The physician may give the 1-hour volume in his order so that the nurse may omit Step 1 and work the problem from Step 2.

    1000 ml D_5W
    1000 ml Ringer's lactate to follow
    1000 ml D_5NS 0.9%
    Run at 125 cc/hr
            Dr. Supersat
    IV set runs 10 gtt/ml

At what flow rate (gtt/min) must this IV be set?

7. The physician orders sodium oxacillin 500 mg IV q4h. The sodium oxacillin has been mixed with 100 ml solution. Administer the solution in 45 minutes. The drop factor is 10 gtt/ml. At what flow rate (gtt/min) must the nurse run this IV?

8. The physician orders Mandol 2 g IV q6h. The Mandol is to be mixed with 100 ml diluent for administration. Administer the solution in 30 minutes. The drop factor is 15 gtt/ml. At what flow rate (gtt/min) must the nurse run this IV?

9. The physician orders 1000 ml D₅W with 10,000 units of heparin added. The patient is to receive 1000 units of heparin per hour. How many milliliters per hour must his IV run?

10. The physician orders 1000 ml D₅W with 20 g MgSO₄ added. The patient is to receive 1 g/hr. How many milliliters per hour must this IV run? The drop factor is 60 gtt/ml. At what flow rate (gtt/min) must the nurse run this IV?

ANSWERS: INTRAVENOUS FLUID RATE CALCULATION

1.

$$\frac{125\ ml}{24\overline{)3000\ ml}} = \text{1-hour volume} = \text{24-hour volume}$$

$$\frac{24}{60}$$
$$\frac{48}{120}$$
$$\frac{120}{}$$

$$\frac{10\ gtt/ml}{60\ min} \times 125\ ml = \text{Flow rate (gtt/min)}$$

$$\frac{\overset{1}{10}}{\underset{6}{60}} \times 125 = \frac{125}{6} = 20\frac{5}{6} \approx 21\ gtt/min$$

2.

$$\frac{150\ ml}{10\overline{)1500\ ml}} = \text{1-hour volume} = \text{10-hour volume}$$

$$\frac{\overset{1}{20}\ gtt/ml}{\underset{3}{60}\ min} \times 150\ ml = \text{Flow rate (gtt/min)}$$

$$\frac{1}{\cancel{3}} \times \cancel{150}^{50} = 50 \text{ gtt/min}$$

3.
$$\begin{array}{r} 10 \text{ ml} \\ 24\overline{)240} \end{array} = \begin{array}{l} \text{1-hour volume} \\ = \text{24-hour volume} \end{array}$$

$$\frac{\cancel{60}^{1} \text{ gtt/ml}}{\cancel{60}_{1} \text{ min}} \times 10 \text{ ml} = 10 \text{ gtt/min}$$

4.
$$\begin{array}{r} 104 \text{ ml} \\ 24\overline{)2500} \text{ ml} \\ \underline{24} \\ 100 \\ \underline{96} \\ 4 \end{array} = \begin{array}{l} \text{1-hour volume} \\ = \text{24-hour volume} \end{array}$$

$$\frac{15 \text{ gtt/ml}}{60 \text{ min}} \times 104 \text{ ml} = \text{Flow rate (gtt/min)}$$

$$\frac{\cancel{15}^{1}}{\cancel{60}_{4}} \times 104 = \frac{104}{4} = 26 \text{ gtt/min}$$

5.
$$\begin{array}{r} 187.5 \text{ ml} \\ 16\overline{)3000.0} \\ \underline{16} \\ 140 \\ \underline{128} \\ 120 \\ \underline{112} \\ 80 \\ \underline{80} \end{array} = \text{16-hour volume}$$

$$\frac{10 \text{ gtt/ml}}{60 \text{ min}} \times 187.5 \text{ ml} = \text{Flow rate (gtt/min)}$$

$$\frac{\cancel{10}^{1}}{\cancel{60}_{6}} \times 187.5 = \frac{187.5}{6} = 31.2 \approx 31 \text{ gtt/min}$$

OR

$$\frac{\overset{1}{\cancel{10}}}{\underset{6}{\cancel{60}}} \times 188 = \frac{188}{6} = 31\frac{1}{3} \approx 31 \text{ gtt/min}$$

6.

$$\frac{10 \text{ gtt/ml}}{60 \text{ min}} \times 125 \text{ ml} = \text{Flow rate (gtt/min)}$$

$$\frac{\overset{1}{\cancel{10}}}{\underset{6}{\cancel{60}}} \times 125 = \frac{125}{6} = 20\frac{5}{6} \approx 21 \text{ gtt/min}$$

7.

$$\frac{\text{Drop factor}}{\text{Time}} \times \text{volume} = \text{Flow rate (gtt/min)}$$

$$\frac{10 \text{ gtt/ml}}{45 \text{ min}} \times 100 \text{ ml} = \frac{1000}{45} = 22\frac{2}{9} \approx 22 \text{ gtt/min}$$

8.

$$\frac{\text{Drop factor}}{\text{Time}} \times \text{volume} = \text{Flow rate (gtt/min)}$$

$$\frac{\overset{1}{\cancel{15}} \text{ gtt/ml}}{\underset{\underset{1}{2}}{\cancel{30}} \text{ min}} \times \overset{50}{\cancel{100}} \text{ ml} = 50 \text{ gtt/min}$$

9. $\dfrac{10,000 \text{ U}}{1000 \text{ ml/hr}} :: \dfrac{1000 \text{ U}}{x \text{ ml/hr}}$

$10,000x = 1,000,000$

$x = 100 \text{ ml/hr}$

$$\frac{\overset{1}{\cancel{1000}} \text{ U/hr}}{\underset{\underset{1}{\cancel{10}}}{\cancel{10,000}} \text{ U}} \times \overset{100}{\cancel{1000}} \text{ ml} = 100 \text{ ml/hr}$$

10. $20 \text{ g}:1000 \text{ ml}::1 \text{ g}:x \text{ ml}$

$20x = 1000$

$x = 50 \text{ ml/hr}$

$$\frac{\cancel{1} \text{ g/hr}}{\underset{1}{\cancel{20}} \text{ g}} \times \overset{50}{\cancel{1000}} \text{ ml} = 50 \text{ ml/hr}$$

$$\frac{60 \text{ gtt/ml}}{60 \text{ min}} \times 50 \text{ ml} = 50 \text{ gtt/min} = \text{IV flow rate}$$

10

Conversion of Temperature Between Fahrenheit and Celsius

The temperature of a patient is one of the physiologic indications of the patient's state of health. A temperature elevation may be an indication that a patient needs antibiotic therapy and/or a drug to lower the temperature. The nurse must keep an accurate record of the patient's temperature. The nurse should be able to convert from the Celsius to the Fahrenheit temperature scale and vice versa.

Originally the term centigrade was used in place of Celsius. Celsius is the metric term and so we will use this term. Five degrees on the Celsius scale equals nine degrees on the Fahrenheit scale. Therefore, the fractions

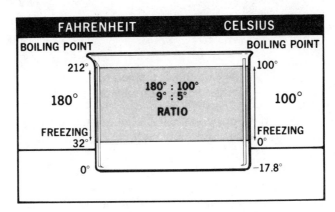

Comparison of Fahrenheit and Celsius temperature scales.

⁵⁄₉ and ⁹⁄₅ are used to convert temperatures from one scale to the other. These fractions indicate the relationship of one scale to the other.

There are a number of formulas that may be used for temperature conversion. I prefer a single formula that can be used to convert either way. I also give one formula to convert from Fahrenheit to Celsius and another to convert from Celsius to Fahrenheit. Choose the method that you find easiest.

FORMULAE FOR TEMPERATURE CONVERSION

Method I

Use the following formula for conversion to either the Fahrenheit or the Celsius scale:

$$\frac{9}{5}°C = °F - 32$$

Because

$$9 \div 5 = 1.8$$

you may use 1.8 instead of ⁹⁄₅:

$$1.8 °C = °F - 32$$

Example 1

Convert 100 °F to °C:

$1.8 °C = °F - 32$
$1.8 °C = 100 - 32$
$1.8 °C = 68$
$$\frac{1.8}{1.8} °C = \frac{68}{1.8}$$
$°C = 37.77$
$°C \approx 37.8$

Convert 37.8 °C to °F:

$1.8 °C = F - 32$
$1.8 \times 37.8 = °F - 32$
$68.04 = °F - 32$
$32 + 68.04 = °F - 32 + 32$
$100.04 = °F$
$100 \approx °F$

Method II

To convert from Fahrenheit to Celsius temperature, subtract 32 from the Fahrenheit temperature and multiply the result by ⁵⁄₉:

$$°C = (°F - 32) \times \frac{5}{9}$$

Note: Remember the difference in the freezing point on the two scales is 32° and the ratio between the scales is 5:9 or ⁵⁄₉.

Example 2

Convert 100 °F to °C.

$$°C = (°F - 32) \times \frac{5}{9}$$

$$°C = (100° - 32) \times \frac{5}{9}$$

$$°C = 68 \times \frac{5}{9}$$

$$°C = \frac{340}{9}$$

$$°C = 37.77 \approx 37.8$$

To convert from Celsius to Fahrenheit temperature, multiply the Celsius temperature by ⁹⁄₅ and then add 32:

$$°F = \left(\frac{9}{5}°C\right) + 32$$

Example 3

Convert 37.8 °C to °F.

$$°F = \left(\frac{9}{5}°C\right) + 32$$

$$°F = \left(\frac{9}{5} \times 37.8\right) + 32$$

$$°F = 68.04 + 32$$

$$°F \approx 100$$

Note: Remember to solve the multiplication within the parentheses first; then finish solving the problem.

PROBLEMS: TEMPERATURE CONVERSION

Convert the following temperatures as indicated. Give answers in decimal form rounded off to the nearest tenth of a degree. Show your work.

1.   37 °C = _____ °F

2. 38.9 °C = _____ °F

3. 36.7 °C = _____ °F

4. 35.8 °C = _____ °F

5.   40 °C = _____ °F

6.   101 °F = _____ °C

7.   97 °F = _____ °C

8.   104 °F = _____ °C

9.   98.8 °F = _____ °C

10.   105 °F = _____ °C

ANSWERS: TEMPERATURE CONVERSION

1.
$$1.8 \ °C = °F - 32$$
$$1.8 \ (37) = °F - 32$$
$$32 + 66.6 = °F - 32 + 32$$
$$98.6 = °F$$

$$°F = \left(\frac{9}{5} \ °C\right) + 32$$
$$°F = \left(\frac{9}{5} \times 37\right) + 32$$
$$°F = \frac{333}{5} + 32$$
$$°F = 66.6 + 32$$
$$°F = 98.6$$

2.
$$1.8 \ °C = °F - 32$$
$$1.8 \ (38.9) = °F - 32$$
$$32 + 70.02 = °F - 32 + 32$$
$$102.02 = °F$$
$$102 \approx °F$$

$$°F = \left(\frac{9}{5} \ °C\right) + 32$$
$$°F = \left(\frac{9}{5} \times 38.9\right) + 32$$
$$°F = \frac{(350.1)}{5} + 32$$
$$°F = 70 + 32$$
$$°F = 102$$

3.
$$1.8 \ °C = °F - 32$$
$$1.8 \ (36.7) = °F - 32$$
$$32 + 66.06 = °F - 32 + 32$$
$$98.06 = °F$$
$$98.1 \approx °F$$

$$°F = \left(\frac{9}{5} \ °C\right) + 32$$
$$°F = \left(\frac{9}{5} \times 36.7\right) + 32$$
$$°F = \frac{(330.3)}{5} + 32$$
$$°F = 66 + 32$$
$$°F = 98.06$$
$$°F \approx 98.1$$

4. $1.8\ °C = °F - 32$
$1.8\ (35.8) = °F - 32$
$32 + 64.44 = °F - 32 + 32$
$96.44 = °F$
$96.4 \approx °F$

$°F = \left(\dfrac{9}{5}\ °C\right) + 32$

$°F = \left(\dfrac{9}{5} \times 35.8\right) + 32$

$°F = \dfrac{322.2}{5} + 32$

$°F = 64.44 + 32$
$°F = 96.44$
$°F \approx 96.4$

5. $1.8\ °C = °F - 32$
$1.8\ (40) = °F - 32$
$32 + 72 = °F - 32 + 32$
$104 = °F$

$°F = \left(\dfrac{9}{5}\ °C\right) + 32$

$°F = \left(\dfrac{9}{5} \times 40\right) + 32$

$°F = \left(\dfrac{360}{5}\right) + 32$

$°F = 72 + 32$
$°F = 104$

6. $1.8\ °C = °F - 32$
$1.8\ °C = 101 - 32$
$1.8\ °C = 69$
$\dfrac{1.8}{1.8}\ °C = \dfrac{69}{1.8}$
$°C = 38.33$
$°C \approx 38.3$

$°C = (°F - 32) \times \dfrac{5}{9}$

$°C = (101 - 32) \times \dfrac{5}{9}$

$°C = 69 \times \dfrac{5}{9}$

$°C = \dfrac{345}{9}$

$°C = 38.3$

7. $1.8\ °C = °F - 32$
$1.8\ °C = 97 - 32$
$1.8\ °C = 65$
$\dfrac{1.8}{1.8}\ °C = \dfrac{65}{1.8}$
$°C = 36.11$
$°C \approx 36.1$

$°C = (°F - 32) \times \dfrac{5}{9}$

$°C = (97 - 32) \times \dfrac{5}{9}$

$°C = 65 \times \dfrac{5}{9}$

$°C = \dfrac{325}{9}$

$°C \approx 36.1$

8. $1.8\ °C = °F - 32$
       $1.8\ °C = 104 - 32$
       $1.8\ °C = 72$
       $\dfrac{1.8\ °C}{1.8} = \dfrac{72}{1.8}$
       $°C = 40$

       $°C = (°F - 32) \times \dfrac{5}{9}$

       $°C = (104° - 32) \times \dfrac{5}{9}$

       $°C = 72 \times \dfrac{5}{9}$

       $°C = \dfrac{360}{9}$

       $°C = 40$

9. $1.8\ °C = F - 32$
       $1.8\ °C = 98.8 - 32$
       $1.8\ °C = 66.8$
       $\dfrac{1.8}{1.8}\ °C = \dfrac{66.8}{1.8}$
       $°C = 37.11$
       $°C \approx 37.1$

       $°C = (°F - 32) \times \dfrac{5}{9}$

       $°C = (98.8 - 32) \times \dfrac{5}{9}$

       $°C = 66.8 \times \dfrac{5}{9}$

       $°C = \dfrac{334}{9}$

       $°C = 37.11$
       $°C \approx 37.1$

10. $1.8\ °C = °F - 32$
       $1.8\ °C = 105 - 32$
       $1.8\ °C = 73$
       $\dfrac{1.8}{1.8}\ °C = \dfrac{73}{1.8}$
       $°C = 40.55$
       $°C \approx 40.6$

       $°C = (°F - 32) \times \dfrac{5}{9}$

       $°C = (105 - 32) \times \dfrac{5}{9}$

       $°C = 73 \times \dfrac{5}{9}$

       $°C = \dfrac{365}{9}$

       $°C = 40.55$
       $°C \approx 40.6$

11

Preparation of Solutions

OBJECTIVES

After completing this chapter, the student will be able to:

1. Define solute, solvent, diluent, solution, percent solution, and ratio strength solution.
2. Calculate the amount of drug necessary to prepare a percent solution from a solid 100 percent drug.
3. Calculate the amount of drug necessary to prepare a percent solution from a 100 percent liquid drug.
4. Calculate the amount of drug necessary to prepare a ratio strength solution from a solid drug.
5. Calculate the amount of drug necessary to prepare a ratio strength solution from a liquid drug.
6. Calculate the amount of a stronger solution necessary to prepare a weaker solution.
7. Calculate the amount of a solvent necessary to prepare any of the above solutions.
8. Determine the strength of a solution, given the amount of drug dissolved in a specific amount of solution.
9. Determine the amount of a given strength solution that may be prepared from a specified amount of drug.
10. Determine the amount of a given strength solution that may be prepared from a specified amount of a stronger solution.
11. Determine the percentage strength of a solution, given the amount of solute and the amount of solution.
12. Define the meaning of percent.
13. Determine the amount of solution needed to give x g of a drug from a percent solution using either formula or ratio and proportion.

METHODS

Nurses and other health care workers may be required to prepare a solution for an irrigation (e.g., vaginal) or a soak (e.g., foot soak). In a large hospital, the pharmacist usually prepares the solution. In small hospitals, nursing homes, or home settings, the nurse may need to prepare a solution or teach a client or the family how to prepare the solution. For example: To protect those who come in contact with persons infected with the HTLV III/LA (AIDS virus) at work or in the home, the United States Public Health Service Centers for Disease Control recommends the use of a freshly prepared solution of sodium hypochlorite (household bleach) in a 1:10 dilution to clean contaminated areas.

The formulas and proportions for calculating the amount of drug needed to prepare a solution are similar to those used for dosage calculations. These formulas and proportions are not hard to understand, but first we need to define several terms.

Solute: Amount of drug or chemical dissolved in a solution.
Solvent: Liquid used to dissolve or dilute the drug or chemical to make a solution (frequently water).
Diluent: Another word for solvent. The definition is the same.

There are several ways to prepare a solution. Some solutions are made from pure (100 percent) drug, whereas other already prepared solutions can be diluted to make weaker solutions. The solution strength may be expressed either as a percentage (for example, a 24 percent solution), which is called a *percent solution*, or as a ratio (for example, a 1:1000 solution), which is called a *ratio strength solution.*

It is necessary to understand percent to understand solutions. When we talk about percent we mean a certain part of the whole, e.g., 10 parts out of every 100 parts of a whole object (50 percent, or one half of the cake was chocolate). Part of a solution is drug; part is solvent.

Remember these important points: Percent means there are x number of parts in every 100 parts. A percent (%) is the same as a fraction in which the denominator is 100; the numerator indicates the part of 100 being considered. For example, a 50 percent solution can be written as a fraction: $50/100$. The 50 represents the amount of drug in the solution and 100 the total solution. It is always a ratio of grams of drug to milliliters of solution. The 50 represents the number of grams of drug being considered. The 100 represents the number of milliliters of solution containing 50 g of drug.

The gram is the weight of 1 milliliter of distilled water at 4 °C.* In other words, a gram of water and a milliliter of water are equivalent. This is the rationale for comparing grams of drug to milliliters of solution in a percentage

---

* Bergersen, Betty S., *Pharmacology in Nursing*, 14th ed. C. V. Mosby Co., St. Louis, 1979, p. 47.

solution. I divide the different types of solutions into sections for ease of discussion. The formula remains the same for each type of solution.

PERCENT SOLUTIONS

Solutions may be made from pure (100 percent) drugs in solid or liquid form. Examples of pure solid drugs are sodium chloride (table salt) and magnesium sulfate (Epsom salt). Examples of a pure liquid drug are cresol or glycerin.

To solve a solution problem you may use either a formula or a ratio and proportion. I personally prefer the ratio and proportion because I can find the solute, the amount of solution or the strength of the solution, without changing the arithmetic process. Both methods are shown; you choose the one you prefer.

Example 1: Using a Liquid Drug

Prepare 1000 ml of a 40 percent cresol solution. Cresol is a pure or 100 percent drug.

We desire 40 percent cresol solution.
We have 100 percent cresol.
We need 1000 ml.

Formula

$$\frac{\text{Desired strength}}{\text{Available strength}} \times \text{Desired amount of solution} = \text{Amount of solute (drug) needed}$$

$$\frac{D}{A} \times \text{Volume desired} = \text{Solute}$$

Step 1: Determine the amount of solute.

$$\frac{D}{A} \times \text{Volume} = \text{Solute}$$

$$\frac{40 \text{ ml}}{\cancel{100} \text{ ml}} \times \overset{10}{\cancel{1000}} \text{ ml} = 400 \text{ ml cresol}$$

We need 400 ml pure cresol to prepare 1000 ml of a 40 percent cresol solution.

Step 2: Determine the amount of solvent. When you are using a liquid drug, you subtract the solute from the amount of solution you desire:

$$1000 \text{ ml solution}$$
$$\underline{-400 \text{ ml cresol}}$$
$$600 \text{ ml solvent}$$

Add 600 ml of solvent to the 400 ml of cresol to obtain 1000 ml of a 40 percent solution.

Ratio–Proportion

Determine the amount of solute.

$$\frac{\text{Desired strength}}{\text{Available strength}} :: \frac{\text{Amount of solute needed}}{\text{Amount of solution}}$$

$$\frac{40 \text{ ml}}{100 \text{ ml}} :: \frac{x \text{ ml}}{1000 \text{ ml}}$$

$$100x = 40,000$$

$$x = 400 \text{ ml}$$

Four hundred milliliters cresol is needed to prepare 1000 ml of a 40 percent solution.

To determine the amount of solvent, proceed as in Step 2 above.

You may wonder why I used milliliters rather than percents in the above example: 40 ml instead of 40 percent and 100 ml instead of 100 percent. Remember when we discussed the meaning of percent we said that we were talking about a part of the whole. In solutions we are talking about the part of a solution that is drug. The part of a solution that is drug is expressed in milliliters in this example because it is a liquid drug (cresol). It would be expressed in grams if the drug were a solid (crystals, powder).

Note: When you are preparing solutions, your formula looks similar to a dosage problem and is solved the same way, but you are not calculating the amount to administer in your answer. You are looking for the *amount of drug or solute* to be dissolved in a solvent to make a solution. Your answer will be in grams of drug (or milliliters of drug, if the solute is a liquid, as in the example above). In the dosage problems, you have been finding *the number of tablets* or *the amount of solution* containing the desired drug dosage.

Example 2: Using a Solid Drug

Prepare 250 ml of a 0.9 percent solution of salt for a gargle.

Step 1: Determine the amount of solute. If you use the formula for this problem, solve as follows:

$$\frac{D}{A} \times V = \text{Solute}$$

$$\frac{0.9 \text{ gm}}{100 \text{ ml}} \times 250 \text{ ml} = 2.25 \text{ g}$$

If you choose the ratio and proportion method to solve this problem, proceed as follows:

$$\frac{\text{Strength desired}}{\text{Strength available}} :: \frac{\text{Amount of solute}}{\text{Amount of solution}}$$

$$\frac{0.9 \text{ g}}{100 \text{ ml}} :: \frac{x \text{ g}}{250 \text{ ml}}$$

$$100x = 225$$

$$x = 2.25 \text{ g}$$

Step 2: Whether you used the formula or the ratio and proportion method, 2.25 g salt is needed to prepare 250 ml of 0.9 percent solution. If salt crystals are to be used, weigh 2.25 g salt. Add it to a measuring graduate and add sufficient water to make 250 ml. Remember a solid drug will take up space in the solution (displacement). You do not know how much space it will take. Always add the solid drug to the mixing container first, then add sufficient solvent to make the desired amount of solution. Tablets of known strength may be used to prepare solutions.

Note: If the preparation to be used is in tablet form instead of crystals, you may need to construct and solve a dosage problem to determine how many tablets to dissolve to make the solution. Assume that the salt for Example 2 comes in 1-g tablets.

To determine the number of tablets needed to make a solution, after the amount of solute has been determined, solve a dosage problem. If you use the formula method, proceed as follows:

$$\frac{D}{H} \times V = \text{Dosage}$$

$$\frac{2.25 \text{ g}}{1 \text{ g}} \times 1 \text{ tab} = 2.25 \text{ tab needed to prepare 250 ml of a}$$
$$0.9 \text{ percent solution}$$

If you prefer the ratio and proportion method, proceed as follows:

$$\text{Strength} : \text{Vehicle} :: \text{Dosage} : \text{Give}$$

$$\frac{1 \text{ g}}{1 \text{ tab}} :: \frac{2.25 \text{ g}}{x \text{ tab}}$$

$$x = 2.25 \text{ tab}$$

Dissolve 2¼ tablets in a small amount of water then add sufficient water to make 250 ml saline gargle.

If you are to instruct a patient how to prepare a saline gargle at home, you could instruct the patient to dissolve ½ teaspoon of salt in an 8-oz glass of warm water and gargle *x* number of times a day as ordered by the physician.

$$1 \text{ tsp} = 4 \text{ to } 5 \text{ ml}$$

$$2.25 \text{ g} = \text{approximately } \frac{1}{2} \text{ teaspoon salt}$$

This is permissible for a gargle but drugs to be taken internally should *NEVER* be approximated.

Exercises: Percent Solutions

Determine the amount of solute and solvent in each of the following exercises.

1. Prepare 500 ml of a 20 percent solution using potassium permanganate crystals.

2. Prepare 250 ml of a 5 percent solution using glycerin, a 100 percent liquid.

3. Prepare 1000 ml of a 10 percent magnesium sulfate solution to use as a soak for an infected finger. Use $MgSO_4$ crystals.

4. Prepare 300 ml of a boric acid solution 0.3 percent using boric acid crystals.

5. Prepare 1 gal of a 25 percent cresol solution.

Answers: Percent Solutions

1.

$$\frac{20 \text{ g}}{\underset{1}{\cancel{100} \text{ ml}}} \times \overset{5}{\cancel{500}} \text{ ml} = 100 \text{ g}$$

$$\frac{20 \text{ g}}{100 \text{ ml}} :: \frac{x \text{ ml}}{500 \text{ ml}}$$
$$100x = 10,000$$
$$x = 100 \text{ g}$$

Weigh 100 g of potassium permanganate and dissolve the crystals in enough water to make 500 ml of solution.

2.

$$\frac{5 \text{ ml}}{\underset{2}{\cancel{100} \text{ ml}}} \times \overset{5}{\cancel{250}} \text{ ml} = \frac{25}{2}$$
$$= 12.5 \text{ ml}$$

$$\frac{5 \text{ ml}}{100 \text{ ml}} :: \frac{x \text{ ml}}{250 \text{ ml}}$$
$$100x = 1250$$
$$x = 12.5 \text{ ml}$$

To determine the amount of solvent, subtract 12.5 ml from the total solution needed:

$$
\begin{array}{r}
250 \text{ ml solution} \\
- \underline{12.5 \text{ ml glycerin}} \\
237.5 \text{ ml solvent}
\end{array}
$$

To prepare 250 ml of a 5 percent solution add 12.5 ml of glycerin and 237.5 ml of solvent (water).

3.

$$\frac{10 \text{ g}}{\underset{1}{\cancel{100} \text{ ml}}} \times \overset{10}{\cancel{1000}} \text{ ml} = 100 \text{ g}$$

$$\frac{10 \text{ g}}{100 \text{ ml}} :: \frac{x \text{ g}}{1000 \text{ ml}}$$
$$100x = 10,000$$
$$x = 100 \text{ g}$$

Weigh 100 g of magnesium sulfate and dissolve in enough water to make 1000 ml.

4.

$$\frac{0.3 \text{ g}}{\underset{1}{\cancel{100} \text{ ml}}} \times \overset{3}{\cancel{300}} \text{ ml} = 0.9 \text{ g}$$

$$\frac{0.3 \text{ g}}{100 \text{ ml}} :: \frac{x \text{ g}}{300 \text{ ml}}$$
$$100x = 90.0$$
$$x = 0.9 \text{ g}$$

Weigh 0.9 g of boric acid crystals and add sufficient water to make 300 ml of solution.

5. 1 gal = 4000 ml

$$\frac{\overset{1}{\cancel{25} \text{ ml}}}{\underset{1}{\underset{\cancel{4}}{\cancel{100} \text{ ml}}}} \times \overset{1000}{\cancel{4000}} \text{ ml} = 1000 \text{ ml cresol}$$

$$\frac{25 \text{ ml}}{100 \text{ ml}} :: \frac{x \text{ ml}}{4000 \text{ ml}}$$
$$100x = 100,000$$
$$x = 1000 \text{ ml}$$

To determine the amount of solvent, subtract 1000 ml from the total solution needed:

$$
\begin{array}{r}
4000 \text{ ml solution} \\
- \underline{1000} \text{ ml cresol} \\
3000 \text{ ml solvent}
\end{array}
$$

Add 1000 ml of cresol to 3000 ml of solvent to make 1 gal of a 25 percent solution.

DILUTING A SOLUTION

Weaker solutions may be made from stronger solutions. Examples of solutions that may be kept as stock drugs in concentrated form are potassium permanganate and benzalkonium chloride. The strength of these solutions may be expressed as a percentage or a ratio.

Example 1:

Prepare 2000 ml of a 6 percent cresol solution from a 10 percent solution. Determine the amount of solute and the amount of solvent. Solve by using the same formula or ratio and proportion that you used to prepare a percentage solution. The desired strength is 6 percent, the available strength is 10 percent. Compare the weaker solution to the stronger solution. You may use the formula:

$$\frac{D}{H} \times \text{Amount of solution} = \text{Amount of solute}$$

Determine the amount of 10 percent cresol needed:

Step 1:
$$\frac{6\%}{10\%} \times 2000 = \text{Amount of solute}$$

$$\frac{6 \text{ ml}}{10 \text{ ml}} \times 2000 \text{ ml} = \frac{12,000}{10} = 1200 \text{ ml}$$

Use 1200 ml of the 10 percent cresol solution to make 2000 ml of a 6 percent cresol solution.

Step 2: Find the amount of solvent to be used:

$$
\begin{array}{r}
2000 \text{ ml solution} \\
- \underline{1200} \text{ ml solute} \\
800 \text{ ml}
\end{array}
$$

Therefore, to make 2000 ml of a 6 percent cresol solution, you add 800 ml water to 1200 ml of the 10 percent cresol solution.

Example 2:

If you prefer the ratio and proportion method, set up the first ratio weaker drug to stronger drug. To prepare a weaker solution from a stronger solution set up the following ratio:

Strength desired (weaker)	:	Strength available (stronger)	::	Amount of solute to use	:	Amount of solution desired

Step 1:

$$D:H \; :: \; solute:solution$$
$$6\%:10\% \; :: \; x \; ml:2000 \; ml$$
$$6 \; ml:10 \; ml \; :: \; x \; ml:2000 \; ml$$
$$10x = 12,000$$
$$x = 1200 \; ml$$

Use 1200 ml of the 10 percent cresol solution to make 2000 ml of a 6 percent cresol solution.

Step 2: Same as above.

Exercises: Diluting a Solution

Determine the amount of solute and the amount of solvent for each of the following exercises.

1. Prepare 200 ml of a 10 percent solution from a 25 percent solution.

2. Prepare 600 ml of an 8 percent solution from a 15 percent solution.

3. Prepare 1500 ml of a 20 percent solution from a 50 percent solution.

4. Prepare 60 ml of a 2 percent solution from a 5 percent solution.

5. Prepare 100 ml of a 5 percent solution from a 25 percent solution.

Answers: Diluting a Solution

1. $\dfrac{10 \text{ ml}}{\overset{}{25} \text{ml}} \times \overset{8}{\cancel{200}} \text{ ml} = 80 \text{ ml}$ $\dfrac{10 \text{ ml}}{25 \text{ ml}} :: \dfrac{x \text{ ml}}{200 \text{ ml}}$

$$25x = 2000$$
$$x = 80 \text{ ml}$$

200 ml solution
$-\underline{80}$ ml solute
120 ml solvent

2. $\dfrac{8 \text{ ml}}{\overset{}{15} \text{ml}} \times \overset{40}{\cancel{600}} \text{ ml} = 320 \text{ ml}$ $\dfrac{8 \text{ ml}}{15 \text{ ml}} :: \dfrac{x \text{ ml}}{600 \text{ ml}}$

$$15x = 4800$$
$$x = 320 \text{ ml}$$

600 ml solution
$-\underline{320}$ ml solute
280 ml solvent

3. $\dfrac{\overset{4}{\cancel{20}} \text{ ml}}{\underset{10}{\cancel{50}} \text{ ml}} \times \overset{150}{\cancel{1500}} \text{ ml} = 600 \text{ ml}$ $\dfrac{20 \text{ ml}}{50 \text{ ml}} :: \dfrac{x \text{ ml}}{1500 \text{ ml}}$

$$50x = 30,000$$
$$x = 600 \text{ ml}$$

1500 ml solution
$-\underline{600}$ ml solute
900 ml solvent

4. $\dfrac{2 \text{ ml}}{\overset{}{5} \text{ml}} \times \overset{12}{\cancel{60}} \text{ml} = 24 \text{ ml}$ $\dfrac{2 \text{ ml}}{5 \text{ ml}} :: \dfrac{x \text{ ml}}{60 \text{ ml}}$

$$5x = 120$$
$$x = 24 \text{ ml}$$

60 ml solution
$-\underline{24}$ ml solute
36 ml solvent

5. $\dfrac{5 \text{ ml}}{\overset{}{25} \text{ml}} \times \overset{4}{\cancel{100}} \text{ ml} = 20 \text{ ml}$ $\dfrac{5 \text{ ml}}{25 \text{ ml}} :: \dfrac{x \text{ ml}}{100 \text{ ml}}$

$$25x = 500$$
$$x = 20 \text{ ml}$$

100 ml solution
$-\underline{20}$ ml solute
80 ml solvent

RATIO STRENGTH SOLUTIONS

Example

Prepare 500 ml of a $1:10,000$ KMnO$_4$ solution from a $1:5000$ solution of KMnO$_4$. This may be solved using fractions or it may be changed to percents.

Solve by using the same formula or ratio and proportion you have been using for solutions.

Using the formula method, we would solve as follows:

Step 1:

$$\frac{D}{A} \times V = \text{Solute}$$

$$\frac{\dfrac{1}{10,000 \text{ ml}}}{\dfrac{1}{5000 \text{ ml}}} \times \frac{500 \text{ ml}}{1} = \frac{\dfrac{500}{10,000}}{\dfrac{1}{5000}}$$

$$\frac{500}{10,000} \div \frac{1}{5000} = \frac{500}{\cancel{10,000}} \times \frac{\overset{1}{\cancel{5000}}}{1} = \frac{500}{2} = 250 \text{ ml}$$

Step 2: Determine the amount of solvent needed.

$$\begin{array}{r} 500 \text{ ml solution desired} \\ -\,250 \text{ ml amount of solute} \\ \hline 250 \text{ ml of water needed} \end{array}$$

Using the ratio–proportion method, we would solve as follows:

Step 1:

$$D \quad : \quad A \quad :: \text{Solute} : \text{Solution}$$

$$\frac{1}{10,000} : \frac{1}{5000} :: x \text{ ml} \; : 500 \text{ ml}$$

$$\frac{1}{5000}\, x = \frac{500}{10,000}$$

$$\frac{1}{5000} \div \frac{1}{5000}\, x = \frac{500}{10,000} \div \frac{1}{5000}$$

$$\frac{\cancel{x}}{\cancel{5000}} \times \frac{\cancel{5000}}{\cancel{x}}\, x = \frac{500}{\cancel{10,000}} \times \frac{\overset{1}{\cancel{5000}}}{1}$$

$$x = \frac{\overset{}{500}}{2}$$

$$x = 250 \text{ ml}$$

Use 250 ml of the 1:5000 solution of $KMnO_4$ to make 500 ml of a 1:10,000 solution of $KMnO_4$.
Done as a percent, you would solve as follows:

$$0.01\%:0.02\%::x \text{ ml}:500 \text{ ml}$$
$$0.02x = 5$$
$$x = \frac{5}{0.02}$$
$$x = 250 \text{ ml}$$

Step 2: To determine the amount of solvent, proceed as in step 2 above.

Exercises: Ratio Strength Solutions

1. Prepare 4 gal of a 1:500 Burow's solution from a 1:250 solution.

2. Prepare 2000 ml of 1:50 potassium permanganate solution from a 1:20 solution.

3. Prepare 125 ml of a 1:25 solution from a 5 percent solution of cresol.

4. Prepare 1000 ml of a 1:5000 solution from a 1:2000 solution.

5. Prepare 500 ml of a 1:750 solution of Zephiran from a 1:250 solution of Zephiran.

Answers: Ratio Strength Solutions

1. *Formula*

$$\frac{\dfrac{1}{500}}{\dfrac{1}{250}} \times 4000 \text{ ml} = \frac{\dfrac{4000}{500}}{\dfrac{1}{250}} = \frac{\overset{2000}{\cancel{4000}}}{\underset{\underset{1}{\cancel{2}}}{\cancel{500}}} \times \frac{\overset{1}{\cancel{250}}}{1} = 2000 \text{ ml}$$

Ratio–Proportion

$$\frac{\dfrac{1}{500}}{\dfrac{1}{250}} \; :: \; \frac{x \text{ ml}}{4000 \text{ ml}}$$

$$\frac{1}{250}\, x = \frac{\overset{8}{\cancel{4000}}}{\underset{1}{\cancel{500}}}$$

$$\frac{\cancel{250}}{1} \times \frac{1}{\cancel{250}}\, x = 8 \times 250$$

$$x = 2000 \text{ ml}$$

4000 ml solution

$-$ 2000 ml solute

2000 ml solvent

Use 2000 ml of 1:250 Burow's solution and 2000 ml solvent to prepare 4000 ml of a 1:500 solution.

2. *Formula*

$$\frac{\dfrac{1}{50}}{\dfrac{1}{20}} \times 2000 \text{ ml} = \frac{\dfrac{2000}{50}}{\dfrac{1}{20}} = \frac{\overset{40}{\cancel{2000}}}{\underset{1}{\cancel{50}}} \times \frac{20}{1} = 800 \text{ ml}$$

Ratio–Proportion

$$\frac{\dfrac{1}{50}}{\dfrac{1}{20}} :: \frac{x \text{ ml}}{2000 \text{ ml}}$$

$$\frac{1}{20} x = \frac{2000}{50}$$

$$x = \frac{2000}{50} \div \frac{1}{20}$$

$$x = \frac{2000}{50} \times \frac{20}{1}$$

$$x = \frac{40,000}{50} = 800 \text{ ml}$$

2000 ml solution
$\underline{-800}$ ml solute
1200 ml solvent

Use 800 ml of 1:20 potassium permanganate and 1200 ml solvent to prepare 2000 ml of a 1:50 solution.

3. *Formula*

$$\frac{\dfrac{1}{25}}{5} \times 125 \text{ ml} = \frac{\dfrac{125}{25}}{5} = \frac{\cancel{125}}{\cancel{25}} \div \frac{5}{1} = \frac{\cancel{5}}{1} \times \frac{1}{\cancel{5}} = 1 \text{ ml}$$

Ratio–Proportion

$$\frac{\dfrac{1}{25}}{5} :: \frac{x \text{ ml}}{125 \text{ ml}}$$

$$5 x = \frac{125}{25}$$

$$\frac{5}{5} x = \frac{125}{25} \div \frac{5}{1}$$

$$x = \frac{125}{25} \times \frac{1}{5}$$

$$x = \frac{125}{125}$$

$$x = 1 \text{ ml}$$

$$\begin{array}{r} 125 \text{ ml solution} \\ \underline{-1} \text{ ml solute} \\ 124 \text{ ml solvent} \end{array}$$

Use 1 ml of 5 percent cresol solution and 124 ml solvent to prepare 125 ml of a 1:25 solution.

4. *Formula*

$$\frac{\dfrac{1}{5000}}{\dfrac{1}{2000}} \times 1000 \text{ ml} = \frac{1000}{5000} \div \frac{1}{2000} = \frac{\overset{1}{\cancel{1000}}}{\cancel{5000}} \times \frac{\overset{400}{\cancel{2000}}}{1} = 400 \text{ ml}$$

Ratio–Proportion

$$\frac{\dfrac{1}{5000}}{\dfrac{1}{2000}} :: \frac{x \text{ ml}}{1000 \text{ ml}}$$

$$\frac{1}{2000} x = \frac{1000}{5000}$$

$$\frac{\cancel{2000}}{1} \times \frac{1}{\cancel{2000}} x = \frac{1000}{\underset{5}{\cancel{5000}}} \times \frac{\overset{2}{\cancel{2000}}}{1}$$

$$x = \frac{2000}{5}$$

$$x = 400 \text{ ml}$$

$$\begin{array}{r} 1000 \text{ ml solution} \\ \underline{-400} \text{ ml solute} \\ 600 \text{ ml solvent} \end{array}$$

Use 400 ml of a 1:2000 solution and 600 ml solvent to prepare 1000 ml of a 1:2000 solution.

5. *Formula*

$$\frac{\dfrac{1}{750}}{\dfrac{1}{250}} \times 500 \text{ ml} = \frac{500}{\underset{3}{\cancel{750}}} \times \frac{1}{\cancel{250}} = \frac{500}{3} = 166.67 \text{ ml} \approx 167 \text{ ml}$$

Ratio–Proportion

$$\frac{\frac{1}{750}}{\frac{1}{250}} :: \frac{x \text{ ml}}{500 \text{ml}}$$

$$\frac{1}{250} x = \frac{500}{750}$$

$$x = \frac{500}{\cancel{750}_{3}} \times \frac{\cancel{250}^{1}}{1}$$

$$x = \frac{500}{3}$$

$$x = 166.67 \text{ ml}$$

$$\begin{array}{r} 500 \text{ ml solution} \\ - 167 \text{ ml solute} \\ \hline 333 \text{ ml solvent} \end{array}$$

Use 167 ml of a 1:250 solution of Zephiran and 333 ml solvent to prepare 500 ml of a 1:750 solution.

DETERMINING THE VOLUME OF A SOLUTION

Sometimes you will know the amount and strength of a solute and need to determine the amount of solution that can be prepared. This type of problem is solved using the same proportion used for other solution problems, the difference being that here the quantity of solution is the unknown factor and the amount and strength of solute is known.

Example

Using 90 ml of cresol, prepare a 5 percent solution. How much solution can be made?

Ratio–Proportion:

Desired : Available :: Amount of : Amount of
strength   strength   solute   solution

$$5\% : \quad 100\% :: \quad 90 \text{ ml} : \quad x \text{ ml}$$
$$5 \text{ ml} : \quad 100 \text{ ml} :: \quad 90 \text{ ml} : \quad x \text{ ml}$$
$$5x = 9000$$
$$x = 1800 \text{ ml of a 5 percent solution can be}$$
made from 90 ml of 100 percent cresol

Formula: We can solve this problem by using the same formula. However, the volume is the unknown quantity. This makes the process of solving the problem more involved.

$$\frac{D}{A} \times \text{Volume} = \text{Amount of solute}$$

$$\frac{5 \text{ ml}}{100 \text{ ml}} \times x \text{ ml} = 90 \text{ ml}$$

$$\frac{5}{100} \div \frac{5}{100} x = 90 \div \frac{5}{100}$$

$$\frac{\cancel{5}}{\cancel{100}} \times \frac{\cancel{100}}{\cancel{5}} x = 90 \times \frac{\overset{20}{\cancel{100}}}{\underset{1}{\cancel{5}}}$$

$$x = 1800 \text{ ml of 5\% solution can be made}$$
$$\text{from 90 ml of 100 percent cresol}$$

Proof:

$$\frac{5 \text{ ml}}{100 \text{ ml}} \times 1800 \text{ ml} = \frac{9000}{100} = 90 \text{ ml}$$

Exercises: Determining the Volume of a Solution

1. Using 4 g of sodium bicarbonate, how much 10 percent solution can you make?

2. Using 50 ml of sodium hypochlorite solution, how many milliliters of a 5 percent solution can you make?

3. Using 60 g of potassium permanganate, how many milliliters of a 25 percent solution can you prepare?

4. Using 9 g of salt, how many milliliters of a 0.9 percent salt solution can you prepare?

5. Using 3 oz hydrogen peroxide, how much 0.5 percent solution can you prepare from a 3 percent solution?

Answers: Determining the Volume of a Solution

1. $\dfrac{10 \text{ g}}{100 \text{ ml}} \times x \text{ ml} = 4 \text{ g}$

   $\dfrac{10}{100} \div \dfrac{10}{100} x = 4 \div \dfrac{10}{100}$

   $\dfrac{\cancel{10}}{\cancel{100}} \times \dfrac{\cancel{100}}{\cancel{10}} x = 4 \times \dfrac{100}{10}$

   $x = \dfrac{400}{10}$

   $x = 40 \text{ ml}$

   $\dfrac{10 \text{ g}}{100 \text{ ml}} :: \dfrac{4 \text{ g}}{x \text{ ml}}$

   $10x = 400$

   $x = 40 \text{ ml}$

A total of 40 ml of a 10 percent sodium bicarbonate solution can be prepared from 4 gm of drug.

2. $\dfrac{5 \text{ ml}}{100 \text{ ml}} \times x \text{ ml} = 50 \text{ ml}$

   $\dfrac{5}{100} \div \dfrac{5}{100} x = 50 \div \dfrac{5}{100}$

   $\dfrac{\cancel{5}}{\cancel{100}} \times \dfrac{\cancel{100}}{\cancel{5}} x = 50 \times \dfrac{100}{5}$

   $x = \dfrac{5000}{5}$

   $x = 1000 \text{ ml}$

   $\dfrac{5 \text{ ml}}{100 \text{ ml}} :: \dfrac{50 \text{ ml}}{x \text{ ml}}$

   $5x = 5000$

   $x = 1000 \text{ ml}$

A total of 1000 ml of a 5 percent sodium hypochlorite solution can be made from 50 ml of drug.

3. $\dfrac{25 \text{ g}}{100 \text{ ml}} \times x \text{ ml} = 60 \text{ g}$

   $\dfrac{25}{100} \div \dfrac{25}{100} x = 60 \div \dfrac{25}{100}$

   $\dfrac{\cancel{25}}{\cancel{100}} \times \dfrac{\cancel{100}}{\cancel{25}} x = 60 \times \dfrac{100}{25}$

   $x = \dfrac{6000}{25}$

   $x = 240 \text{ ml}$

   $\dfrac{25 \text{ g}}{100 \text{ ml}} :: \dfrac{60 \text{ g}}{x \text{ ml}}$

   $25x = 6000$

   $x = 240 \text{ ml}$

A total of 240 ml of a 25 percent solution of potassium permanganate can be made from 60 g of drug.

4.
$$\frac{0.9 \text{ g}}{100 \text{ ml}} \times x \text{ ml} = 9 \text{ g}$$

$$\frac{0.9}{100} \div \frac{0.9}{100} x = 9 \div \frac{0.9}{100}$$

$$\frac{\cancel{0.9}}{\cancel{100}} \times \frac{\cancel{100}}{\cancel{0.9}} x = 9 \times \frac{100}{0.9}$$

$$x = \frac{900}{0.9}$$

$$x = 1000 \text{ ml}$$

$$\frac{0.9 \text{ g}}{100 \text{ ml}} :: \frac{9 \text{ g}}{x \text{ ml}}$$

$$0.9x = 900$$

$$x = 1000 \text{ ml}$$

A total of 1000 ml of 0.9 percent salt solution can be made from 9 g salt.

5. 3 oz = 90 ml

$$\frac{0.5 \text{ ml}}{3 \text{ ml}} \times x \text{ ml} = 90 \text{ ml}$$

$$\frac{0.5}{3} \div \frac{0.5}{3} x = 90 \div \frac{0.5}{3}$$

$$\frac{\cancel{0.5}}{\cancel{3}} \times \frac{\cancel{3}}{\cancel{0.5}} x = 90 \times \frac{3}{0.5}$$

$$x = \frac{270}{0.5}$$

$$x = 540 \text{ ml}$$

$$\frac{0.5 \text{ ml}}{3 \text{ ml}} :: \frac{90 \text{ ml}}{x \text{ ml}}$$

$$0.5x = 270$$

$$x = 540 \text{ ml}$$

A total of 540 ml of 0.5 percent hydrogen peroxide solution can be made from 3 oz of a 3% solution.

DETERMINING THE PERCENT OF A SOLUTION

Nurses frequently state that they do not need to know how to prepare solutions. The pharmacist does it for them. However, there are dangers inherent in such an attitude. A nursing drug paper presented a story, reprinted from JAMA, about a baby brought into the hospital unable to breathe because the mucous membranes of her nose were swollen, cutting off her breath, causing acute nasal obstruction and respiratory distress. The mother had been instructed to make saline nose drops to use in the baby's nose. When the mother was questioned, it was found she had prepared the nose drops by using 1 tablespoon of salt to 8 oz of water.*

* Ulin, I.S., Bartlett, G.: Iatrogenic acute nasal obstruction in an obligate nose breather. JAMA 243:1657 (April 25) 1980.

To determine the percent of the solution prepared by the mother in this report, set up a proportion using the known quantities. The mother added 1 tbs of salt to an 8-oz glass of warm water.

Known Facts: 1 tbs = 15 ml

1 g of a drug is equal to 1 ml of water at 4°C

A percent solution is the number of grams of drug in 100 ml of solution.

8 oz = 240 ml

From these facts we can set up a proportion:

$$\frac{x \text{ g}}{100 \text{ ml}} = \frac{15 \text{ g}}{240 \text{ ml}}$$

$$240x = 1500$$

$$x = 6.25 \text{ gm}$$

Place the value of *x* over 100 and change to a percent:

$$\frac{6.25 \text{ g}}{100 \text{ ml}} = 0.0625 = 6.25 \text{ percent}$$

The mother had prepared a 6.25 percent solution. She should have prepared a 0.5 percent solution by using ¼ teaspoon of salt to an eight ounce glass of water. Regardless of why she prepared a dangerously concentrated solution, nurses are frequently the ones who are responsible for teaching patients/clients how to prepare similar kinds of solutions. It is of the utmost importance that nurses be able to instruct others correctly and/or be able to prepare a solution in the correct strength. Nurses may not prepare solutions frequently, but they should be able to prepare them correctly when necessary.

Exercises: Determining the Percent of a Solution

1. If 90 g of drug is used to prepare 500 ml of a solution, what is the percentage strength of this solution?

2. If 240 g of drug is used to prepare 750 ml of solution, what is the percentage strength of this solution?

3. If 60 ml of drug is used to prepare 240 ml of solution, what is the percentage strength of this solution?

4. If 200 ml of drug is used to prepare 4000 ml of solution, what is the percentage strength of this solution?

5. If 1 g of drug is used to prepare 1000 ml of solution, what is the percentage strength of this solution?

Answers: Determining the Percent of a Solution

1. $\dfrac{x \text{ g}}{100 \text{ ml}} \times 500 \text{ ml} = 90 \text{ g}$

$$\dfrac{x}{100} \times \dfrac{\overset{1}{\cancel{500}}}{\underset{1}{\cancel{500}}} = \dfrac{90}{500}$$

$$\dfrac{x}{\underset{1}{\cancel{100}}} \times \overset{1}{\cancel{100}} = 0.18 \times 100$$

$$x = 18 \text{ g}$$

$$\dfrac{18 \text{ g}}{100 \text{ ml}} = 0.18 = 18 \text{ percent solution}$$

$\dfrac{x \text{ g}}{100 \text{ ml}} :: \dfrac{90 \text{ g}}{500 \text{ ml}}$

$$500x = 9000$$

$$x = 18 \text{ g}$$

2. $\dfrac{x \text{ g}}{100 \text{ ml}} \times 750 \text{ ml} = 240 \text{ g}$

$$\dfrac{x}{100} \times \dfrac{\overset{1}{\cancel{750}}}{\underset{1}{\cancel{750}}} = \dfrac{240}{750}$$

$$\dfrac{x}{100} = 0.32$$

$$\dfrac{x}{\underset{1}{\cancel{100}}} \times \overset{1}{\cancel{100}} = 0.32 \times 100$$

$$x = 32 \text{ g}$$

$$\dfrac{32 \text{ g}}{100 \text{ ml}} = 0.32 = 32 \text{ percent solution}$$

$\dfrac{x \text{ g}}{100 \text{ ml}} :: \dfrac{240 \text{ g}}{750 \text{ ml}}$

$$750x = 24{,}000$$

$$x = 32 \text{ g}$$

3. $\dfrac{x \text{ ml}}{100 \text{ ml}} \times 240 \text{ ml} = 60 \text{ ml}$

$$\dfrac{x}{100} \times \dfrac{\overset{1}{\cancel{240}}}{\underset{1}{\cancel{240}}} = \dfrac{60}{240}$$

$$\dfrac{x}{\underset{1}{\cancel{100}}} \times \overset{1}{\cancel{100}} = 0.25 \times 100$$

$$x = 25 \text{ ml}$$

$$\dfrac{25}{100} = 0.25 = 25 \text{ percent solution}$$

$\dfrac{x \text{ ml}}{100 \text{ ml}} :: \dfrac{60 \text{ ml}}{240 \text{ ml}}$

$240x = 6000$

$x = 25 \text{ ml}$

4. $\dfrac{x \text{ ml}}{100 \text{ ml}} \times 4000 \text{ ml} = 200 \text{ ml}$

$$\dfrac{x}{100} \times \dfrac{\overset{1}{\cancel{4000}}}{\underset{1}{\cancel{4000}}} = \dfrac{\overset{5}{\cancel{200}}}{\underset{100}{\cancel{4000}}}$$

$$\dfrac{x}{\cancel{100}} \times \cancel{100} = 0.05 \times 100$$

$$x = 5 \text{ ml}$$

$$\dfrac{5}{100} = 0.05 = 5 \text{ percent solution}$$

$\dfrac{x \text{ ml}}{100 \text{ ml}} :: \dfrac{200 \text{ ml}}{4000 \text{ ml}}$

$4000x = 20,000$

$x = 5 \text{ ml}$

5. $\dfrac{x \text{ g}}{100 \text{ ml}} \times 1000 \text{ ml} = 1 \text{ g}$

$$\dfrac{x}{100} \times \dfrac{\overset{1}{\cancel{1000}}}{\underset{1}{\cancel{1000}}} = \dfrac{1}{1000}$$

$$\dfrac{x}{\underset{1}{\cancel{100}}} \times \overset{1}{\cancel{100}} = 0.001 \times 100$$

$$x = 0.1 \text{ g}$$

$$\dfrac{0.1}{100} = 0.001 = 0.1 \text{ percent solution}$$

$\dfrac{x \text{ g}}{100 \text{ ml}} :: \dfrac{1 \text{ g}}{1000 \text{ ml}}$

$1000x = 100$

$x = 0.1 \text{ g}$

PREPARATION OF A DOSAGE FROM A PERCENT SOLUTION

Occasionally it is necessary to derive or check a dosage from a percent solution.

Set up a dosage problem using the percent of the solution as the drug available and 100 ml as the vehicle. Work the dosage problem by formula or ratio and proportion.

Example

Give 10 g $MgSO_4$ from a 50 percent solution.

Formula

$$\frac{D}{H} \times V = G$$

$$\frac{10 \text{ g}}{50 \text{ g}} \times 100 \text{ ml} = \frac{1000}{50} = 20 \text{ ml}$$

Ratio–Proportion

$$\frac{50 \text{ g}}{100 \text{ ml}} :: \frac{10 \text{ g}}{x \text{ ml}}$$

$$50x = 1000$$

$$x = 20 \text{ ml}$$

Whichever method we use, we find that 20 ml of solution contains 10 g $MgSO_4$.

Note: Remember 50 percent means there is 50 g of drug in 100 ml of solution.

Exercises: Preparation of a Dosage from a Percent Solution

1. Prepare 2 g chloral hydrate from a 25 percent solution.

2. Give 6 g $MgSO_4$ from a 15 percent solution.

3. Give 40 g of drug from a 70 percent solution.

4. Give 25 g of drug from a 30 percent solution.

5. Add 2 g lidocaine to 800 ml D_5W. You have a 1 percent solution. How much 1 percent solution will you add?

Answers: Preparation of a Dosage from a Percent Solution

1. $$\frac{2 \text{ g}}{25 \text{ g}} \times 100 \text{ ml} = \frac{200}{25}$$
$$= 8 \text{ ml}$$

$$\frac{25 \text{ g}}{100 \text{ ml}} :: \frac{2 \text{ g}}{x \text{ ml}}$$
$$25x = 200$$
$$x = 8 \text{ ml}$$

Use 8 ml chloral hydrate solution to obtain 2 g chloral hydrate.

2. $$\frac{6 \text{ g}}{15 \text{ g}} \times 100 \text{ ml} = \frac{600}{15}$$
$$x = 40 \text{ ml}$$

$$\frac{15 \text{ g}}{100 \text{ ml}} :: \frac{6 \text{ g}}{x \text{ ml}}$$
$$15x = 600$$
$$x = 40 \text{ ml}$$

Use 40 ml $MgSO_4$ solution to obtain 6 g $MgSO_4$.

3. $$\frac{40 \text{ g}}{70 \text{ g}} \times 100 \text{ ml} = \frac{4000}{70}$$
$$x = 57.1 \approx 57 \text{ ml}$$

$$70 \text{ g}:100 \text{ ml} :: 40 \text{ g}:x \text{ ml}$$
$$70 x = 4000$$
$$x = 57.1 \approx 57 \text{ ml}$$

Use 57 ml solution to obtain 40 g of drug.

4. $$\frac{25 \text{ g}}{30 \text{ g}} \times 100 \text{ ml} = \frac{2500}{30}$$
$$x = 83\frac{1}{3} \approx 83 \text{ ml}$$

$$\frac{30 \text{ g}}{100 \text{ ml}} :: \frac{25 \text{ g}}{x \text{ ml}}$$
$$30 x = 2500$$
$$x = 83\frac{1}{3} \text{ ml} \approx 83 \text{ ml}$$

Use 83 ml solution to obtain 25 g of drug.

5. $$\frac{2 \text{ g}}{1 \text{ g}} \times 100 \text{ ml} = 200 \text{ ml}$$

$$\frac{1 \text{ g}}{100 \text{ ml}} :: \frac{2 \text{ g}}{x \text{ ml}}$$
$$x = 200 \text{ ml}$$

Use 200 ml of 1 percent lidocaine to obtain 2 g lidocaine.

PROBLEMS: SOLUTION PREPARATION

1. Prepare 1000 ml physiologic saline 0.9 percent using 1 g salt tablets.

2. Prepare 500 ml of a 10 percent solution of boric acid from crystals.

3. Using 1 oz of a 2 percent hydrogen peroxide solution prepare a 1 percent solution. How much solution will this make?

4. Prepare 1 liter of 1:1000 potassium permanganate solution from a 1:500 potassium permanganate solution.

5. You are told to give 10 ml of a 10 percent solution. If you give this amount, how do you know it is equal to 1 g of drug—the amount ordered by the physician?

6. Prepare 1 pint of a 2 percent solution from 250-mg tablets.

7. How much solution can be made using 30 ml of a drug in a 5 percent solution.

8. Prepare 400 ml of a ½ percent solution from a 5 percent solution.

9. Prepare 2 gal of a 15 percent solution of cresol from pure cresol.

10. Prepare 800 ml of a 25 percent solution of $MgSO_4$ solution from $MgSO_4$ crystals.

11. How much 10 percent solution would be needed to make 1 gal of a 3 percent solution? How much water would be needed?

12. How much of a 5 percent solution would be needed to prepare 1500 ml of a 2 percent solution? How much water would be needed?

13. How much of a 1:5 stock solution would be needed to prepare 1 L of a 1:20 solution? How much water would be needed?

14. How much of a 1:2000 solution would be needed to prepare 4000 ml of a 1:10,000 solution? How much water would be needed?

15. How much vinegar is necessary to make 1000 ml of a 4 percent solution? How much water would be needed?

16. If 30 g of drug is used to prepare 1000 ml of solution, what is the percentage strength of this solution?

17. If 250 ml of glycerin is used to prepare 4000 ml of solution, what is the percentage strength of this solution?

18. Add 1 g of lidocaine to 100 ml of IV solution, using a 2 percent lidocaine solution. How much of the 2 percent solution will you need to add to the IV to equal 1 g?

19. How much sodium hypochlorite (household bleach) is needed to prepare 1 gallon of a 1:10 solution? How much water?

ANSWERS: SOLUTION PREPARATION

1. *Step 1:* Determine amount of salt:

$$\frac{0.9 \text{ g}}{\underset{1}{\cancel{100} \text{ ml}}} \times \overset{10}{\cancel{1000}} \text{ ml} = 9 \text{ g}$$

OR

$$\frac{0.9 \text{ g}}{100 \text{ ml}} :: \frac{x \text{ g}}{1000 \text{ ml}}$$
$$100x = 900$$
$$x = 9 \text{ g}$$

Step 2: Determine the number of tablets needed to obtain 9 g salt:

$$\frac{9 \text{ g}}{1 \text{ g}} \times 1 \text{ tab} = 9 \text{ tab}$$

OR

$$1 \text{ g} : 1 \text{ tab} :: 9 \text{ g} : x \text{ tab}$$
$$\frac{1 \text{ g}}{1 \text{ tab}} :: \frac{9 \text{ g}}{x \text{ tab}}$$
$$x = 9 \text{ tab}$$

Dissolve 9 tablets of salt in enough water to make 1000 ml of solution.

2.

$$\frac{10 \text{ g}}{\underset{1}{\cancel{100} \text{ ml}}} \times \overset{5}{\cancel{500}} \text{ ml} = 50 \text{ g}$$

OR

$$10 \text{ g}:100 \text{ ml}::x \text{ g}:500 \text{ ml}$$
$$100x = 5000$$
$$x = 50 \text{ g}$$

Weigh 50 g of boric acid crystals and dissolve them in enough water to make 500 ml of solution.

3.   1 oz = 30 ml of 2 percent hydrogen peroxide solution.

$$\frac{1 \text{ ml}}{2 \text{ ml}} \times x \text{ ml} = 30 \text{ ml}$$

$$\frac{1}{2} \div \frac{1}{2} \times x \text{ ml} = 30 \div \frac{1}{2}$$

$$\frac{\cancel{1}}{\cancel{2}} \times \frac{\cancel{2}}{\cancel{1}} \times x \text{ ml} = 30 \times \frac{2}{1}$$

$$x = 60 \text{ ml}$$

OR

$$1 \text{ ml}:2 \text{ ml}::30 \text{ ml}:x \text{ ml}$$
$$x = 60 \text{ ml}$$

60 ml of 1 percent hydrogen peroxide solution can be made from 30 ml of a 2 percent solution.

4. Remember that values must be in the same unit of measure. You must convert liters to milliliters: 1 L = 1000 ml.

$$\frac{\dfrac{1}{1000}}{\dfrac{1}{500}} \times 1000 \text{ ml} = \frac{\dfrac{1000}{1000}}{\dfrac{1}{500}}$$

$$= \frac{1000}{1000} \div \frac{1}{500}$$

$$= \frac{\overset{1}{\cancel{1000}}}{\underset{1}{\cancel{1000}}} \times \frac{500}{1}$$

$$= 500 \text{ ml KMnO}_4$$

OR

$$\frac{1}{1000 \text{ ml}} : \frac{1}{500 \text{ ml}} :: x \text{ ml} : 1000 \text{ ml}$$

$$\frac{1}{500} x = \frac{1000}{1000}$$

$$\frac{1}{500} \div \frac{1}{500} x = \frac{1000}{1000} \div \frac{1}{500}$$

$$\frac{1}{\cancel{500}} \times \frac{\cancel{500}}{1} x = \frac{\cancel{1000}}{\cancel{1000}} \times \frac{500}{1}$$

$$x = 500 \text{ ml KMnO}_4$$

5. Check by using a solution problem:

$$\frac{10 \text{ g}}{100 \text{ ml}} \times 10 \text{ ml} = \frac{100}{100} = 1 \text{ g}$$

Set up a ratio and proportion to check it:

$$10 \text{ g} : 100 \text{ ml} :: x \text{ g} : 10 \text{ ml}$$
$$100x = 100$$
$$x = 1 \text{ g}$$

You would be correct to give 10 ml.
Remember, a ratio and proportion may be used to find any part of the proportion if you know the other three values.

6. 1 pt = 500 ml

Step 1: Determine amount of drug needed:

$$\frac{2 \text{ g}}{\cancel{100} \text{ ml}} \times \cancel{500}^{\,5} \text{ ml} = 10 \text{ g}$$

OR

$$2 \text{ g} : 100 \text{ ml} :: x \text{ g} : 500 \text{ ml}$$

$$\frac{2 \text{ g}}{100 \text{ ml}} :: \frac{x \text{ g}}{500 \text{ ml}}$$

$$100x = 1000$$

$$x = 10 \text{ g}$$

Step 2: Solve a dosage problem to determine how many 250-mg tablets are needed. Convert 10 g to milligrams: 10 g = 10,000 mg.

$$\frac{\overset{40}{\cancel{10,000}} \text{ mg}}{\underset{1}{\cancel{250} \text{ mg}}} \times 1 \text{ tab} = 40 \text{ tab}$$

Dissolve 40 tablets in sufficient water to make 1 pt of solution.

7.
$$\frac{5 \text{ ml}}{100 \text{ ml}} \times V = 30 \text{ ml}$$

$$\frac{5}{100} \div \frac{5}{100} V = 30 \div \frac{5}{100}$$

$$\frac{\cancel{5}}{\cancel{100}} \times \frac{\cancel{100}}{\cancel{5}} V = 30 \times \frac{100}{5}$$

$$V = \overset{6}{\cancel{30}} \times \frac{100}{\underset{1}{\cancel{5}}}$$

$$V = 600 \text{ ml of solution can be made.}$$

OR

$$5 \text{ ml} : 100 \text{ ml} :: 30 \text{ ml} : x \text{ ml}$$
$$5x = 3000$$
$$x = 600 \text{ ml of solution}$$

8. *Step 1:* Determine the amount of drug needed. Convert ½ percent to a decimal:

$$\frac{1}{2}\% = 2\overline{)1.0}^{\,0.5\%}$$

$$\frac{0.5\%}{\underset{1}{\cancel{5}\%}} \times \overset{80}{\cancel{400}} \text{ ml} = 40.0 \text{ ml of drug}$$

OR

$$\frac{0.5\%}{5\%} :: \frac{x \text{ ml}}{400 \text{ ml}}$$
$$5x = 200.0$$
$$x = 40 \text{ ml of drug}$$

Step 2: Determine the amount of solvent:

$$
\begin{array}{r}
400 \text{ ml solution desired} \\
40 \text{ ml drug needed} \\
\hline
360 \text{ ml water needed}
\end{array}
$$

Add 40 ml of drug and 360 ml water to prepare 400 ml of a ½% solution from a 5% solution.

9. *Step 1:* 2 gal = 8000 ml

$$\frac{15}{\underset{1}{\cancel{100}}} \times \overset{80}{\cancel{8000}} \text{ ml} = 1200 \text{ ml pure cresol}$$

OR

$$15 \text{ ml}:100 \text{ ml}::x \text{ ml}:8000 \text{ ml}$$
$$100x = 120,000$$
$$x = 1200 \text{ ml pure cresol}$$

Step 2:

$$
\begin{array}{r}
8000 \text{ ml cresol solution desired} \\
- 1200 \text{ ml pure cresol} \\
\hline
6800 \text{ ml water needed to prepare the solution}
\end{array}
$$

Add 1200 ml of cresol and 6800 ml water to prepare 8000 ml of a 15% cresol solution.

10. *Step 1:*

$$\frac{25 \text{ g}}{\underset{1}{\cancel{100} \text{ ml}}} \times \overset{8}{\cancel{800}} \text{ ml} = 200 \text{ g}$$

OR

$$\frac{25 \text{ g}}{100 \text{ ml}} :: \frac{x \text{ g}}{800 \text{ ml}}$$
$$100x = 20,000$$
$$x = 200 \text{ g}$$

Step 2: Add 200 g of $MgSO_4$ crystals to a measuring graduate and add sufficient water to make 800 ml of solution.

11. *Step 1:*

$$\frac{3 \text{ ml}}{\underset{1}{\cancel{10} \text{ ml}}} \times \overset{400}{\cancel{4000}} \text{ ml} = 1200 \text{ ml}$$

OR

$$3 \text{ ml}:10 \text{ ml}::x \text{ ml}:4000 \text{ ml}$$
$$10x = 12,000$$
$$x = 1200 \text{ ml}$$

Step 2:

4000 ml solution desired

<u>1200</u> ml of 10% solution needed

2800 ml water needed

Add 1200 ml of 10 percent solution and 2800 ml of water to prepare 4000 ml of a 10% solution.

12. *Step 1:*

$$\frac{2 \text{ ml}}{\underset{1}{\cancel{5} \text{ ml}}} \times \overset{300}{\cancel{1500}} \text{ ml} = 600 \text{ ml of 5 percent solution}$$

OR

$$2 \text{ ml}:5 \text{ ml}::x \text{ ml}:1500 \text{ ml}$$
$$5x = 3000$$
$$x = 600 \text{ ml of 5 percent solution}$$

Step 2:

1500 ml solution desired

<u>−600</u> ml of 5 percent solution

900 ml water needed

13. *Step 1:*

$$\frac{\dfrac{1}{20}}{\dfrac{1}{5}} \times 1000 = \frac{\dfrac{1000}{20}}{\dfrac{1}{5}} = \frac{1000}{\underset{4}{\cancel{20}}} \times \frac{\overset{1}{\cancel{5}}}{1} = \frac{1000}{4} = 250 \text{ ml}$$

OR

$$1:20 = 0.05;\ 1:5 = 0.2$$

$$0.05\ \text{ml}:0.2\ \text{ml}::x\ \text{ml}:1000\ \text{ml}$$
$$0.2x = 5000\ \text{ml}$$
$$x = 250\ \text{ml}$$

Step 2:

$$\begin{array}{r} 1000\ \text{ml solution needed} \\ -\,250\ \text{ml of 1:5 solution} \\ \hline 750\ \text{ml water needed} \end{array}$$

Add 250 ml of a 1:5 solution and 750 ml of water to prepare 1000 ml of a 1:20 solution.

14. *Step 1:*

$$\frac{\dfrac{1}{10,000}}{\dfrac{1}{2000}} \times 4000\ \text{ml} = \frac{\dfrac{4000}{10,000}}{\dfrac{1}{2000}}$$

$$= \frac{\overset{800}{\cancel{4000}}}{\cancel{10,000}} \times \frac{\overset{1}{\cancel{2000}}}{1} = 800\ \text{ml of 1:2000 solution}$$
$$\underset{1}{\cancel{5}}$$

OR

$$1:10,000 : 1:2000 :: x\ \text{ml}:4000\ \text{ml}$$

$$\frac{1}{2000}\,x = \frac{4000}{10,000}$$

$$\frac{1}{2000} \div \frac{1}{2000}\,x = \frac{4000}{10,000} \div \frac{1}{2000}$$

$$\frac{\cancel{1}}{\cancel{2000}} \times \frac{\cancel{2000}}{\cancel{1}}\,x = \frac{\overset{800}{\cancel{4000}}}{\cancel{10,000}} \times \frac{\overset{1}{\cancel{2000}}}{1}\,x = 800\ \text{ml of 1:2000 solution}$$
$$\underset{1}{\cancel{5}}$$

Step 2:

4000 ml solution needed
 800 ml of 1:2000 solution
3200 ml water needed

Add 800 ml of 1:2000 solution and 3200 ml water to prepare 4000 ml of a 1:10,000 solution.

15. *Step 1:*

$$\frac{4 \text{ ml}}{\underset{1}{\cancel{100} \text{ ml}}} \times \cancel{1000}^{10} \text{ ml} = 40 \text{ ml vinegar}$$

OR

$$4 \text{ ml}:100 \text{ ml}::x \text{ ml}:1000 \text{ ml}$$
$$100x = 4000 \text{ ml}$$
$$x = 40 \text{ ml vinegar}$$

Step 2:

1000 ml solution needed
  40 ml vinegar
 960 ml water needed

Add 40 ml of vinegar and 960 ml water to prepare 1000 ml of a 4 percent vinegar solution.

16.

$$\frac{x \text{ g}}{100 \text{ ml}} \times 1000 \text{ ml} = 30 \text{ g}$$

$$\frac{x}{\underset{1}{\cancel{100}}} \times \cancel{100}^{1} \times \frac{\cancel{1000}^{1}}{\underset{1}{\cancel{1000}}} = \frac{30 \times 100}{1000} = \frac{3000}{1000}$$

$$x = 3 \text{ g}$$

OR

$$\frac{x \text{ g}}{100 \text{ ml}} \; :: \; \frac{30 \text{ g}}{1000 \text{ ml}}$$

$$1000x = 3000$$

$$x = 3 \text{ g of drug per 100 ml}$$

$$\frac{3 \text{ g}}{100 \text{ ml}} = 100\overline{)3.00}^{0.03} = 3 \text{ percent solution}$$

17.

$$\frac{x \text{ ml}}{100 \text{ ml}} \times 4000 \text{ ml} = 250 \text{ ml}$$

$$\frac{x}{\cancel{100}} \times \cancel{100}^{1} \times \frac{\cancel{4000}^{1}}{\cancel{4000}_{1}} = \frac{250 \times 100}{4000}$$

$$x = \frac{25,000}{4000}$$

$$x = 6.25 \text{ ml}$$

OR

$$\frac{x \text{ ml}}{100 \text{ ml}} \; :: \; \frac{250 \text{ ml}}{4000 \text{ ml}}$$

$$4000x = 25,000$$

$$x = 6.25 \text{ ml}$$

$$\frac{6.25 \text{ ml}}{100 \text{ ml}} = 100\overline{)6.2500}^{0.0625} = 6.25 \text{ percent solution}$$

18.

$$\frac{1 \text{ g}}{2 \text{ g}} \times 100 \text{ ml} = \frac{100}{2} = 50 \text{ ml of 2 percent lidocaine solution}$$

OR

$$2 \text{ g} : 100 \text{ ml} :: 1 \text{ g} : x \text{ ml}$$

$$2x = 100$$

$$x = 50 \text{ ml of 2 percent lidocaine solution}$$

19.   1 gal = 4000 ml   1 ml:10 ml::x ml:4000 ml

$$\frac{1 \text{ ml}}{\cancel{10} \text{ ml}} \times \cancel{4000}^{400} \text{ ml} = 400 \text{ ml}$$

10 x = 4000

x = 400 ml

$$\begin{array}{r} 4000 \text{ ml} \\ -400 \text{ ml} \\ \hline 3600 \text{ ml} \end{array}$$

Add 400 ml sodium hypochlorite and 3600 ml of water to prepare 4000 ml of sodium hypochlorite solution.

12

Apothecaries' System

OBJECTIVES

After completing this chapter, the student will be able to:

1. Name the basic measures used in the apothecaries' system for weight and for volume.
2. Read and interpret the abbreviations for apothecaries' symbols and numbers.
3. Write the symbols and the correct dosage using Roman numerals.
4. Convert from one apothecaries' measure to another.

The apothecaries' system of weights and measures was brought to America from England by the first colonists. The apothecary shop sold herbs and other medicines to cure the ills of humankind. This system of weights has been used by pharmacists to prepare medications throughout our history. Today, however, the metric system is rapidly becoming the universal system of weights and measures, and has largely replaced the apothecaries' system in the United States.

Drug and pharmaceutical companies now use the metric system of weights and measures in labeling their products. The label of drugs that were originally produced under the apothecaries' system still state the apothecaries' equivalent on the label, in addition to the metric equivalent. Examples of these older drugs are codeine, phenobarbital, atropine, and aspirin, to name only a few. Many physicians, trained in the apothecaries' system of measurement, still write orders under this system. However, until all drugs are ordered in the metric system, nurses must learn both the metric and apothecaries' systems.

APOTHECARIES' SYSTEM UNITS OF VOLUME AND WEIGHT

In the apothecaries' system the basic unit of weight is the grain. Originally the grain was equal in weight to a grain of wheat. The next largest measurement is the scruple, which, since it is not used in medicine, is not discussed here. The next largest measurement is the dram. The dram is used in both liquid and solid measurement. One dram is equal to 60 grains. There are eight drams in the next largest measure, which is the ounce. In order of increasing size, the ounce is followed by the pint, the quart, and the gallon. There are 12 ounces in an apothecaries' pound, in contrast with the avoirdupois pound familiar to most people which contains 16 ounces.

The basic unit of volume is the minim. The minim is approximately equal to the amount of water that would weigh 1 grain. The fluid dram, the fluid ounce, the pint, the quart, and the gallon are the other units of volume, listed in order of increasing size.

The symbol for minim is ℳ
The symbol for grain is gr
The symbol for dram is ℨ (The dram is smaller than the ounce—the symbol is smaller)
The symbol for ounce is ℥ (The ounce is larger than the dram—the symbol is larger)
O is the symbol for pint and comes from the Latin octarius, meaning ⅛ of a gallon
C comes from the Latin word conguis meaning the container for 1 gallon.

When apothecaries' symbols are used, the amount is expressed in Roman numerals. The Roman numeral may be written in lower case numerals. They are written after the apothecaries' symbol.

ℨ iv   = 4 drams
ℳ iii   = 3 minims
gr v   = 5 grains
℥ xxx = 30 ounces
O i   = 1 pint

Fractions are expressed in Arabic numerals. The fraction is written after the apothecaries' symbol, for example, gr ¼. The symbol for ½ is ss. It comes from the Latin word *semis*, meaning one half. Thus: gr ss = ½ grain and gr viiss = 7½ grains. Dots are placed above the bar to distinguish a lowercase i, meaning 1, from a lowercase "el," which stands for 50.

If Arabic numerals are used in place of Roman numerals the Arabic numeral is written in front of the apothecaries' term, for example, 6 grains. The only exception to this rule is a fraction, which is always written after the apothecaries' symbol, for example, gr ½; gr ¼.

APOTHECARIES' EQUIVALENT TABLE

Units of Volume	Equivalents
60 minims (m̃ lx)	= 1 fluid dram (f𝔷i)
8 fluid drams (f𝔷 viii)	= 1 ounce (f℥i)
16 fluid ounces (f℥ xvi)	= 1 pint (pt i or O i)
2 pints (O ii)	= 1 quart (qt i)
32 fluid ounces (f℥ xxxii)	= 1 quart (qt i)
4 quarts	= 1 gallon (gal i or C i)

Units of Weight	Equivalents
60 grains (gr lx)	= 1 dram (𝔷 i)
8 drams (𝔷 viii)	= 1 ounce (℥ i)
12 ounces (℥ xii)	= 1 pound (lb i)

To measure liquids in the apothecaries' system use a minim glass or a medicine glass marked with the apothecaries' measurements. If you do not have a minim glass to measure small amounts of drugs, a minim/cc syringe may be used to measure the amount accurately.

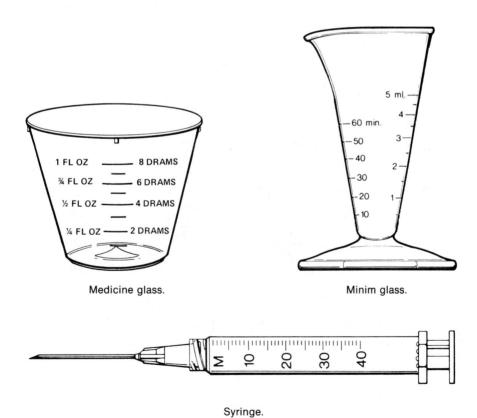

Medicine glass.

Minim glass.

Syringe.

PROBLEMS: APOTHECARIES' SYSTEM

1. *Read the following for practice.*

♏ xviiss _____	f ℨ iv _____
ℨ vii _____	gr ss _____
℥ xv _____	f ℥ ix _____
gr i _____	gr ¹/₃₀₀ _____

2. *Write the following in apothecaries' notations.*

Eleven ounces _____	One half fluid ounce _____
4½ drams _____	2 fluid drams _____
1 pint _____	One hundred forty minims _____
7 gallons _____	Two quarts _____

3. *Equivalents.*

1 qt	= _____ pt		ℨ iv	= _____ gr
♏ xxx	= _____ f ℨ		℥ iss	= _____ ℨ
gr lx	= _____ ℨ		C i	= _____ O
ℨ viii	= _____ ℥		O iv	= _____ qt
f ℥ xvi	= _____ O		pt iii	= _____ f ℥
♏ xc	= _____ f ℨ		f ℥ ii	= _____ f ℨ
ℨ ii	= _____ gr		gr xxx	= _____ ℨ
f ℥ ivss	= _____ f ℨ		lb iss	= _____ ℥ (troy)
½ gal	= _____ qt		120 gr	= _____ ℨ
O x	= _____ gal		pt iiss	= _____ ℥

ANSWERS: APOTHECARIES' SYSTEM

1.

♏ xviiss	17½ minims		f ℨ iv	4 fluid drams
ℨ vii	7 drams		gr ss	½ grain
℥ xv	15 ounces		f ℥ ix	9 fluid ounces
gr i	1 grain		gr ¹/₃₀₀	¹/₃₀₀ grain

2.

Eleven ounces	℥ xi	One half fluid ounce	f ℥ ss
4½ drams	ℨ ivss	2 fluid drams	f ℨ ii
1 pint	1 pt or O i	One hundred forty minims	♏ cxl
7 gallons	C vii	Two quarts	2 qt

3.

1 qt	=	2	pt	ʒ iv	=	240	gr
♏ xxx	=	½	fʒ	℥ iss	=	12	ʒ
gr lx	=	1	ʒ	C i	=	8	O
ʒ viii	=	1	℥	O iv	=	2	qt
f℥ xvi	=	1	O	pt iii	=	48	fʒ
♏ xc	=	1½	fʒ	f℥ ii	=	16	fʒ
ʒ ii	=	120	gr	gr xxx	=	½	ʒ
f℥ ivss	=	36	fʒ	lb iss	=	18	℥ (troy)
½ gal	=	2	qt	120 gr	=	2	ʒ
O x	=	1¼	gal	pt iiss	=	40	℥

13

Household System

The household system is used for administering medication in the home. It is also used in determining patient oral intake from the food tray or water pitcher. The intake is then converted to the metric equivalent. This system is not a complete system because it contains only units of volume. The units are the glass, cup, tablespoon, teaspoon, and drop. There is a lack of standardization in the size of these utensils, so the size may vary considerably.

A drop varies in size depending on the temperature of the liquid, the viscosity of the liquid, the angle at which the dropper is held, and the diameter of the bore of the dropper. Drops and minims are thought to be equivalent, but because of the variations in drop sizes they should never be used interchangeably.

The teaspoon varies in size from 4 to 5 ml or more. The American Standards Institute sets the standard for an American teaspoon at 5 ml. For household measurements, 3 teaspoons equal 1 tablespoon.

If a medication is to be measured by the household system, the physician must order the drug in household measures. If the patient's condition, the potency of the drug, or other factors require greater accuracy of measurement, the nurse may help the patient to secure the appropriate calibrated measuring equipment.

Memorize the following equivalents (accepted standards):

60 drops (gtt) = 1 teaspoon (t or tsp)
2 teaspoons = 1 dessertspoon (Dssp)
3 teaspoons = 1 tablespoon (T, Tbs or Tbsp)
2 tablespoons = 1 ounce (oz)
6 fluid ounces = 1 teacup
8 fluid ounces = 1 glass
16 ounces = 1 pound

Pints and quarts are found in the home but these are considered apothecaries' measures.

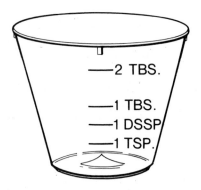

Example

The patient drank 4½ glasses of water. How many ounces did he drink?

To solve this problem, multiply the number of glasses by the number of ounces in one glass:

$$1 \text{ glass} = 8 \text{ ounces}$$

$$8 \text{ oz} \times 4\frac{1}{2} \text{ glasses} = 36 \text{ oz}$$

or set up a ratio:

$$\frac{1 \text{ glass}}{8 \text{ oz}} = \frac{4\frac{1}{2} \text{ glasses}}{x \text{ oz}}$$

$$1\,x = 36 \text{ oz}$$

Exercises: Household System

1. A patient drank six 4-oz cups of juice. How many ounces did he drink?

2. How many tablespoons are in 8 oz?

3. How many teaspoons are in 90 drops of a liquid?

4. You are to calculate a patient's fluid intake: She had a teacup of coffee, a 4-oz glass of juice, and a glass of milk. How many ounces of fluid did this patient drink?

5. Calculate the day's intake of fluid for Mr. Aron.

   Breakfast
   Juice: 4 oz container
   Teacup of coffee

   Lunch
   Coke: 8 oz

   Dinner
   Juice: 4 oz
   Glass of milk

Answers: Household System

1. $6 \times 4\ oz = 24\ oz$

2. $8\ oz \times 2\ Tbsp = 16\ Tbsp$

3. $90\ drops \div 60\ drops = 1\frac{1}{2}\ tsp$

4.   6 oz coffee
       4 oz juice
     $\underline{+8\ oz\ milk}$
      18 oz total intake

5.   4 oz juice
6 oz coffee
8 oz Coke
4 oz juice
+8 oz milk
30 oz total intake

PROBLEMS: EQUIVALENTS

1. 6 t   = _____ T

2. 18 t   = _____ oz

3. 4 oz   = _____ T

4. 12 oz   = _____ cups

5. 12 oz   = _____ glasses

6. 4 T   = _____ oz

7. 1 glass = _____ oz

8. 3 cups   = _____ oz

ANSWERS: EQUIVALENTS

1. 6 t   = __2__ T

2. 18 t   = __3__ oz

3. 4 oz   = __8__ T

4. 12 oz   = __2__ cups

5. 12 oz   = __1½__ glasses

6. 4 T   = __2__ oz

7. 1 glass = __8__ oz

8. 3 cups   = __18__ oz

14

Conversion Among the Apothecaries', Household, and Metric Systems

OBJECTIVES

After completing this chapter, the student will be able to:

1. State the ratio for conversion between grains and grams.
2. Solve problems to convert grains to grams.
3. Solve problems to convert grams to grains.
4. State the ratio for conversion between milligrams and grains.
5. Solve problems to convert milligrams to grains.
6. Solve problems to convert grains to milligrams.
7. State the ratio for conversions of milliliters and minims.
8. Solve problems to convert milliliters to minims.
9. Solve problems to convert minims to milliliters.
10. State the ratio for conversion between ounces and milliliters.
11. Solve problems to convert ounces to milliliters.
12. Solve problems to convert milliliters to ounces.
13. Explain the inequivalence of the apothecaries' and metric systems.

Medications that have been in use for many years list both the metric and apothecaries' equivalents on the label. Examples include ferrous sulfate, phenobarbital, nitroglycerin, and codeine, to name only a few. The two systems are only approximately equivalent, so you will see discrepancies on the labels. One grain in the apothecaries' system is equal to 0.0648 g. The accepted approximate metric equivalent is 60, 64, or 65 mg depending on how the number is rounded off. For example, you may have an order for 300 mg ferrous sulfate and the preparation stocked is marked 325 mg. Both 300 mg and 325 mg equal 5 gr. Request that the physician write the order according to the strength supplied in the hospital. If the order is written as 5 gr, either strength (above) is correct.

$$60 \text{ mg} \times 5 \text{ gr} = 300 \text{ mg}$$

$$64 \text{ mg} \times 5 \text{ gr} = 320 \text{ mg}$$

$$65 \text{ mg} \times 5 \text{ gr} = 325 \text{ mg}$$

To convert from milligrams to grains or grains to milligrams, in this book we will use the ratio 1 gr:60 mg.

Convert 5 gr to milligrams

$$60 \text{ mg}:1 \text{ gr}::x \text{ mg}:5 \text{ gr}$$

$$1x = 300 \text{ mg}$$

Convert 300 mg to grains

$$60 \text{ mg}:1 \text{ gr}::300 \text{ mg}:x \text{ gr}$$

$$60x = 300$$

$$\frac{60}{60} x = \frac{300}{60}$$

$$x = 5 \text{ gr}$$

To convert from grams to grains, or grains to grams, in this book we will use the ratio 15 gr:1 g. Remember that conversions from one system to another are only approximate equivalents.

Convert 60 gr to grams

$$15 \text{ gr}:1 \text{ g}::60 \text{ gr}:x \text{ g}$$

$$15x = 60$$

$$\frac{15}{15} x = \frac{60}{15}$$

$$x = 4 \text{ g}$$

Convert 4 g to grains

$$15 \text{ gr}:1 \text{ g}::x \text{ gr}:4 \text{ g}$$

$$x = 60 \text{ gr}$$

EQUIVALENTS

Apothecaries' System	Metric Equivalent	Approximate Metric Equivalents Used By Nurses
1 gr	0.0648 g	60 or 64 or 65 mg
15.432 gr	1 g	1 g
1 minim	0.06161 ml	0.06 ml
60 minims	3.697 ml	4 ml
1 dram	3.697 ml	4 ml
8 drams	29.5729 ml	30 ml
16 ounces = 1 pint	473.167 ml	500 ml or ½ L
2 pints = 1 quart	946.333 ml	1000 ml or 1 L

Below and on the following pages are examples of drugs labeled with different milligram–grain equivalences. These differences underscore the fact that the apothecaries' and the metric systems are not equal but are approximate equivalents. Be very careful when giving drugs ordered in one system and supplied in another system of measurement. Small differences in some drugs may produce harmful effects.

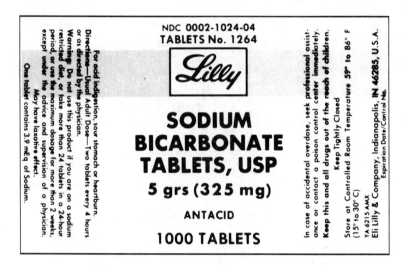

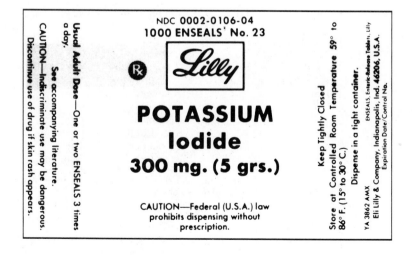

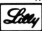

SACCHARIN SODIUM TABLETS, USP
1/2 gr (32 mg)

NDC 0002-1021-04
1000   TABLETS No. 1222

USE OF THIS PRODUCT MAY BE HAZARDOUS TO YOUR HEALTH. THIS PRODUCT CONTAINS SACCHARIN WHICH HAS BEEN DETERMINED TO CAUSE CANCER IN LABORATORY ANIMALS.

Keep Tightly Closed

YA 4826 AMX
ELI LILLY AND COMPANY
INDIANAPOLIS, IN 46285, U.S.A.
Expiration Date/Control No.

One tablet is equivalent in sweetening power to two teaspoonsful of sugar.
Store at Controlled Room Temperature 59° to 86°F (15° to 30°C)

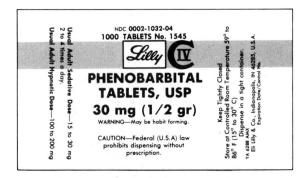

PHENOBARBITAL TABLETS, USP
30 mg (1/2 gr)

NDC 0002-1032-04
1000 TABLETS No. 1545

WARNING—May be habit forming.

CAUTION—Federal (U.S.A) law prohibits dispensing without prescription.

Usual Adult Sedative Dose—15 to 30 mg
2 to 4 times a day.
Usual Adult Hypnotic Dose—100 to 200 mg

Keep Tightly Closed
Store at Controlled Room Temperature 59° to 86° F (15° to 30° C)
Dispense in a tight container.
YA 6288 AMX
Eli Lilly & Co. Indianapolis, IN 46285, U.S.A.
Expiration Date/Control No.

COMPARISON OF THE THREE SYSTEMS OF MEASURE

Metric		Apothecaries'		Household[a]
Volume	Weight	Volume	Weight	Volume
0.06 ml	0.06 g or 60 mg	1 minim (m i)	1 grain (gr i)	1 drop (1 gtt)
1 ml	1 g	15 or 16 minims	15 or 16 grains	
4–5 ml	4 g	1 fluid dram (fʒ i)	1 dram (ʒ i)	1 tsp[b]
15–16 ml[c]	15–16 g[c]	4 fluid drams (fʒ iv)	4 drams (ʒ iv)	1 Tbs
30–32 ml[d]	30–32 g[d]	1 fluid ounce (fʒ i)	1 ounce(ʒ i)	2 Tbs
180 ml		6 ounces (fʒ vi)		1 cup
240 ml		8 ounces (fʒ viii)		1 glass
0.5 L or 500 ml[e]		16 ounces or 1 pt (O i)		1 pint
1 L or 1000 ml[f]	1 kg	32 ounces or 1 qt	2.2 lb avoirdupois	1 quart

[a] The household system is inaccurate and should not be used for medications unless the drug is specifically ordered in household measurement.
[b] A scant teaspoon = 4 ml; a full teaspoon = 5 ml.
[c] One-half ounce is usually considered to be 15 ml.
[d] One ounce is usually considered to be 30 ml.
[e] Pints are not exactly equal to 500 ml but this is the accepted standard used in nursing.
[f] Quarts are not exactly equal to 1000 ml but this is the accepted standard used in nursing.

APPROXIMATE EQUIVALENTS THAT NURSES SHOULD MEMORIZE[a]

Metric	Apothecaries'	Household
Weight		
0.06 g or 60 mg	1 grain	
1 g	15 or 16 grains	
1 kg	2.2 lb (avoirdupois)	
Volume		
0.06 ml	1 minim	
1 ml	15–16 minims	
4 ml	1 dram	1 scant tsp
15 ml	½ ounce	1 Tbs
30 ml	8 drams	
30 ml	1 ounce	6 or 8 tsp
30 ml	1 ounce	2 Tbs
180 ml	6 ounces	1 cup
240 ml	8 ounces	1 glass
500 ml or 0.5 L	1 pint	
500 ml or 0.5 L	16 ounces	
1000 ml or 1 L	32 ounces	
1000 ml or 1 L	1 quart	
4000 ml or 4 L	1 gallon	

[a] Remember the two ratios described earlier: 1 gr:60 mg and 15 gr:1 g.

Exercises: Conversion from Metric Units to Apothecaries' Units

1. 15 ml   = f℥   _____

2. 10 ml   = f℈   _____

3. 24 ml   = f℈   _____

4. 750 mg   = gr   _____

5. 300 mg   = gr   _____

6. 0.25 g   = gr   _____

7. 0.5 ml   = ♏   _____

8. 0.2 ml   = ♏   _____

9. 30 mg   = gr   _____

10. 10 mg   = gr   _____

11. 3 ml   = ♏   _____

12. 1 ml   = ♏   _____

13. 60 ml   = f℥   _____

14. 1500 ml   = O   _____

15. 500 ml   = qt   _____

Answers: Conversion from Metric Units to Apothecaries' Units

1.	15 ml	=	f℥ ss
2.	10 ml	=	f℈ iiss
3.	24 ml	=	f℈ vi
4.	750 mg	=	gr xii
5.	300 mg	=	gr v
6.	0.25 g	=	3¾ gr
7.	0.5 ml	=	♏ viiss
8.	0.2 ml	=	♏ iii
9.	30 mg	=	gr ss
10.	10 mg	=	gr ⅙
11.	3 ml	=	♏ xlv
12.	1 ml	=	♏ xv
13.	60 ml	=	f℥ ii
14.	1500 ml	=	O iii
15.	500 ml	=	½ qt

Exercises: Conversion from Apothecaries' Units to Metric Units

1.	♏ xv	=	_____ ml
2.	℈ iii	=	_____ ml
3.	℥ iv	=	_____ ml
4.	gr xxx	=	_____ g
5.	gr x	=	_____ mg
6.	O iv	=	_____ L
7.	C v	=	_____ L
8.	♏ cxx	=	_____ ml
9.	gr iss	=	_____ mg
10.	O iiss	=	_____ ml
11.	℈ xii	=	_____ ml

12. ʒ xvi   = _____ ml

13. gr xv   = _____ mg

14. gr viiss   = _____ g

15. gr ⅓   = _____ mg

Answers: Conversion from Apothecaries' Units to Metric Units

1. ♏ xv   = ___1___ ml

2. ʒ iii   = ___12___ ml

3. ʒ iv   = ___120___ ml

4. gr xxx   = ___2___ g

5. gr x   = ___600___ mg

6. O iv   = ___2___ L

7. C v   = ___20___ L

8. ♏ cxx   = ___8___ ml

9. gr iss   = ___90___ mg

10. O iiss   = ___1250___ ml

11. ʒ xii   = ___48___ ml

12. ʒ xvi   = ___480___ ml

13. gr xv   = ___1000___ mg

14. gr viiss   = ___0.5___ g

15. gr ⅓   = ___20___ mg

PROBLEMS: CONVERSION AMONG MEASURING SYSTEMS

Conversion Between Metric and Apothecaries' Systems

1. The physician orders gr v of ferrous sulfate. You have ferrous sulfate in 325-mg tablets.

2. The physician orders phenobarb gr ¼. You have phenobarb in 16-mg tablets.

3. The physician orders ephedrine gr ⅜. You have ephedrine in 23-mg tablets.

4. The physician orders atropine gr 1/100. You have atropine in 0.65-mg tablets.

5. The physician orders colchicine gr 1/100. You have colchicine in 0.6 mg tablets.

6. The physician orders thyroid 0.03 g. You have thyroid in gr ss tablets.

7. The physician orders codeine gr ss. You have codeine in 15-mg tablets.

8. The physician orders seconal 0.1 g. You have seconal in gr iss capsules.

9. The physician orders atropine 200 mcg. You have atropine sulfate as gr 1/150 per milliliter.

10. The physician orders morphine sulfate gr ⅛. You have morphine sulfate as 8 mg/ml.

11. The physician orders phenobarbital 45 mg. You have phenobarbital in gr ½ tablets.

12. The physician orders aspirin gr iiss. You have aspirin in 300-mg tablets.

Conversion Between Metric and Household Systems

You are to teach patients to take their medicine at home as given in the hospital. Convert each of the following instructions from the metric to the household systems:

1. The patient is to take her potassium supplement in at least 120 ml of orange juice. How many ounces of orange juice should she use?

2. Alister has been receiving 5 ml of Ceclor for an infection. His mother is to continue giving the medication at home. How many teaspoons of medication should she give?

3. Mr. Norris is to take 10 ml of Triaminicol cough medicine every 4 hours as necessary for his cough. How many teaspoons should he take per dose?

4. Anna, a child, is to receive 250 mg Ilosone liquid. How many teaspoons of liquid should she receive if the Ilosone comes as 125 mg per 5 ml?

5. Mrs. Johnson is to prepare a vinegar douche using 15 ml vinegar. How many tablespoons of vinegar will she use? She must put the vinegar in 500 ml water. Roughly, how many teacups? How many glasses? Using an apothecary item found in the home, how many pints?

6. Mrs. Harris has been told to limit her fluid intake to 800 ml/day. How many 8-oz glasses of fluid may she have?

7. Mr. Smith is to prepare a 50% hydrogen peroxide solution using 30 ml hydrogen peroxide. How many teaspoons of hydrogen peroxide should he use? How many tablespoons? An equal amount of water must be measured in the same manner.

8. Mr. Jones has been having diarrhea. The physician wants him to take 60 ml Kaopectate. How many tablespoons of Kaopectate should Mr. Jones take? How many teaspoons is this?

ANSWERS

Conversion Between Metric and Apothecaries' Systems

1.

$$1 \text{ gr} : 60 \text{ mg} :: 5 \text{ gr} : x \text{ mg} \qquad\qquad 1 \text{ gr} : 65 \text{ mg} :: 5 \text{ gr} : x \text{ mg}$$

$$x = 300 \text{ mg} \qquad\qquad\qquad\qquad x = 325 \text{ mg}$$

Both answers are correct. You may give the 325-mg tablet.

2.

$$1 \text{ gr} : 60 \text{ mg} :: \text{gr } \frac{1}{4} : x \text{ mg}$$

$$x = \frac{60}{4}$$

$$x = 15 \text{ mg}$$

If we had used 64 mg = 1 gr

$$1 \text{ gr} : 64 \text{ mg} :: \text{gr } \frac{1}{4} : x \text{ mg}$$

$$x = \frac{64}{4}$$

$$x = 16 \text{ mg}$$

Both answers are correct.
You may use the 16-mg tablet to equal gr ¼.

3.

$$1 \text{ gr} : 60 \text{ mg} :: \text{gr } \frac{3}{8} : x \text{ mg}$$

$$x = \frac{180}{8}$$

$$x = 22.5 \approx 23 \text{ mg}$$

Give the 23-mg tablet of ephedrine.

4.

$$1 \text{ gr}:60 \text{ mg} :: \text{gr} \frac{1}{100} : x \text{ mg}$$

$$x = \frac{60}{100}$$

$$x = 0.60 \text{ mg}$$

Had you used 1 gr:65 mg instead, gr $\frac{1}{100}$ would have equaled 0.65 mg.

Give one 0.65-mg tablet of atropine.

5.

$$1 \text{ gr}:60 \text{ mg} :: \text{gr} \frac{1}{100} : x \text{ mg}$$

$$1x = \frac{60}{100}$$

$$x = 0.6 \text{ mg}$$

Give one 0.6-mg tablet of colchicine.

6.

$$15 \text{ gr}:1 \text{ g} :: x \text{ gr}:0.03 \text{ g}$$

$$1x = 0.45$$

$$x = \frac{45}{100} = \frac{9}{20} = 0.45 \approx \frac{1}{2} \text{ gr}$$

0.03 g = 30 mg

$$1 \text{ gr}:60 \text{ mg} :: x \text{ gr}:30 \text{ mg}$$

$$60x = 30$$

$$x = \frac{30}{60} = \frac{1}{2} \text{ gr}$$

Give one ½-grain tablet of thyroid.

7.

$$1 \text{ gr}:60 \text{ mg} :: \text{gr} \frac{1}{2} : x \text{ mg}$$

$$1x = \frac{60}{2}$$

$$x = 30 \text{ mg}$$

Give 2 tablets of codeine 15 mg: 15 mg × 2 tab = 30 mg = gr ss.

8.

$$15 \text{ gr}:1 \text{ g}::x \text{ gr}:0.1 \text{ g}$$

$$1x = 1.5 \text{ gr}$$

$$x = 1\frac{1}{2} \text{ gr}$$

Give one 1½-grain capsule of seconol.

9. 200 mcg $= 0.2$ mg

1 gr $= 60$ mg

$$1 \text{ gr}:60 \text{ mg}::\text{gr} \frac{1}{150} :x \text{ mg}$$

$$x = \frac{\overset{6}{\cancel{60}}}{\underset{15}{\cancel{150}}}$$

$$x = 0.4 \text{ mg (or 400 mcg)}$$

After converting gr ¹⁄₁₅₀ to 0.4 mg, set up and solve a dosage problem to determine how much atropine sulfate solution to give.

$$\frac{\overset{1}{\cancel{0.2 \text{ mg}}}}{\underset{2}{\cancel{0.4 \text{ mg}}}} \times 1 \text{ ml} = \frac{1}{2} = 0.5 \text{ ml}$$

Give 0.5 ml of atropine

10.

$$1 \text{ gr}:60 \text{ mg}::x \text{ gr}:8 \text{ mg}$$

$$60x = 8$$

$$x = \frac{8}{60}$$

$$= \frac{2}{15} \text{ gr}$$

Had you used 1 gr:64 mg the fraction would have equaled ⁸⁄₆₄ = ⅛ gr. Give 1 ml of morphine sulfate, as it contains 8 mg (= gr ⅛).

11.

$$60 \text{ mg}:1 \text{ gr}::x \text{ mg}:\text{gr } \frac{1}{2}$$

$$x = \frac{1}{2} \times 60$$

$$x = 30 \text{ mg}$$

$$\frac{45 \text{ mg}}{30 \text{ mg}} \times 1 \text{ tab} = 1\frac{1}{2} \text{ tab}$$

12.

$$60 \text{ mg}:1 \text{ gr}::300 \text{ mg}:x \text{ gr}$$

$$60x = 300$$

$$x = 5 \text{ gr}$$

$$\frac{2.5 \text{ gr}}{5 \text{ gr}} \times 1 \text{ tab} = \frac{1}{2} \text{ tab}$$

Conversion Between Metric and Household Systems

1. $30 \text{ ml} = 1 \text{ oz}$ $\dfrac{30 \text{ ml}}{1 \text{ oz}} = \dfrac{120 \text{ ml}}{x \text{ oz}}$

   $120 \text{ ml} \div 30 \text{ ml/oz} = 4 \text{ oz}$

$$30x = 120$$

$$x = 4 \text{ oz}$$

The patient should use a measuring cup marked in ounces.

2. $5 \text{ ml} = 1 \text{ tsp}$

The mother should administer 1 tsp of Ceclor.

3. $5 \text{ ml} = 1 \text{ tsp}$

$$\frac{1 \text{ tsp}}{5 \text{ ml}} = \frac{x \text{ tsp}}{10 \text{ ml}}$$

$$5x = 10$$

$$x = 2 \text{ tsp}$$

Mr. Norris should take 2 tsp of Triaminicol.

4.

$$\frac{\overset{2}{\cancel{250}\text{ mg}}}{\underset{1}{\cancel{125}\text{ mg}}} \times 1 \text{ tsp} = 2 \text{ tsp}$$

$$\frac{125 \text{ mg}}{1 \text{ tsp}} :: \frac{250 \text{ mg}}{x}$$

$$125x = 250$$

$$x = 2 \text{ tsp}$$

$$5 \text{ ml} = 1 \text{ tsp}$$
$$10 \text{ ml} = 2 \text{ tsp}$$

Anna should receive 2 teaspoons of Ilosone.

5. 15 ml = 1 Tbs or 3 tsp vinegar

500 ml = 1 pint (16 oz)

$$= 2\frac{3}{4} \text{ teacups (6 oz) (495 ml)}$$

$$= 2 \text{ glasses (8 oz) (480 ml)}$$

Conversion factors are not really equivalent. Household conversion factors vary. Mrs. Johnson could also use the following household items to measure the water:

$$2 \text{ measuring cups (250 ml)} = 500 \text{ ml}$$
$$1 \text{ pint jar} = 500 \text{ ml}$$

and use 1 tablespoon or 3 teaspoons to measure the vinegar.

6. Convert ounces to milliliters:

$$8 \text{ oz} \times 30 \text{ ml/oz} = 240 \text{ ml}$$

Determine how many 240-ml glasses Mrs. Harris may drink:

$$240\overline{)800 \text{ ml}}^{\,3.33} = 3\frac{1}{3} \text{ glasses of fluid}$$
$$\underline{720}$$
$$800$$
$$\underline{720}$$
$$800$$
$$\underline{720}$$

7.   30 ml = 6 tsp

                               30 ml = 2 Tbs

Mr. Smith can use 6 teaspoons or 2 tablespoons to measure both the hydrogen peroxide and the water.

8. Convert milliliters to tablespoons: 15 ml = 1 Tbs

$$\frac{15 \text{ ml}}{1 \text{ Tbs}} :: \frac{60 \text{ ml}}{x \text{ Tbs}}$$

$$15x = 60$$

$$x = 4 \text{ Tbs of Kaopectate}$$

Convert milliliters to teaspoons: 5 ml = 1 tsp

$$\frac{5 \text{ ml}}{1 \text{ tsp}} :: \frac{60 \text{ ml}}{x \text{ tsp}}$$

$$5x = 60$$

$$x = 12 \text{ tsp of Kaopectate}$$

15

Computerization of Drug Records

OBJECTIVES

After completing this chapter, the student will be able to:

1. Recognize the components of a computer printout.
2. Read the time from the twenty-four-hour clock.
3. Write the time of day using the twenty-four-hour clock.

To simplify the enormous job of record keeping, hospital pharmacies are converting to a computerized system. As the medication orders are sent to the pharmacy, the pharmacist will add the new drugs to the computer listing and delete the drugs that have been discontinued. A medication sheet containing all current drugs ordered for the patient will be sent to the patient's nursing unit each day. This system will save the nursing unit time that was formerly spent transcribing medication orders to a kardex or medication cards.

Included on the printout sheet will be all of the patient's medications, dose, frequency of administration, route, and times of administration. The computerized medication sheet will have the advantages of containing more detailed information and greater consistency and accuracy than the systems currently in use in most hospitals.

Look at the computer printout sheet.

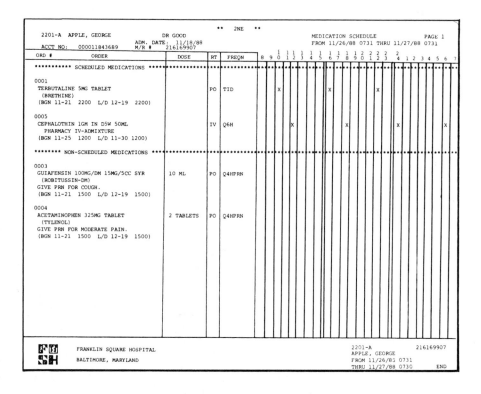

The top of the sheet contains the patient's name, hospital number, and other information pertinent to identification, the inclusive date, and the time period that the sheet represents.

In the left-hand column, ORD# is the number of the physician's order. Each order written will have a sequenced number (activity orders, laboratory tests, diet, medications, etc.), making it easier to refer back to the chart and the medication order in question.

Under "order," there may be a listing of the drug by both generic and proprietary name, the time the medication was started, and the time of the last dose to be given.

					Times 1 1 1 1 8 9 0 1 2 3 4
Order #	**Order**	**Dose**	**Rt**	**Freqn**	
0001	Terbutaline	5 mg	Po	Tid	X

BGN 11/21 2200 L/D 12/19 2200
(Begin) (Date) (Time) (Last (Date) (time)
                              dose)

Each hospital will decide on the format to be used by that hospital.

The nurse must learn to tell time by the 24-hour clock in order to use these medication sheets.

Study the 24-hour clock.

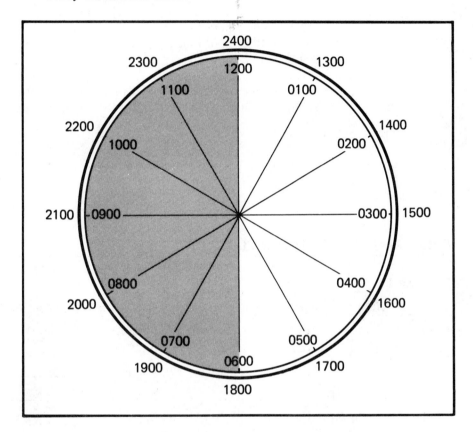

The numbers inside the clock represent the hours from 1 AM until 12 noon. The numbers on the outside of the clock represent the time from 1 PM until midnight.

To tell time read the numbers inside the clock as follows: 0100 hours, 1 AM; 0200 hours, 2 AM; and so on around the clock until 1200 hours, 12 noon. Then moving along the outside, read as follows: 1300 hours, 1 PM; 1400 hours, 2 PM; and finally 2400 hours, 12 midnight. Thus 1325 hours, or thirteen hundred twenty-five hours, would be 1:25 PM.

The time from 12 midnight to 1 AM is stated as 0001, 0002, 0005, 0010, 0015, 0030, 0045, etc, that is, only minutes are stated.

To convert from traditional time to 24-hour time, for time between 1 PM and midnight simply add 12 hours to the traditional time and delete the colon used in traditional time (for time between 12 midnight and 12 noon simply delete the colon, e.g., 10:00 AM = 1000 hours). For example:

1:00 PM + 1200 = 1300 24-hour time
2:10 PM + 1200 = 1410 24-hour time
7:45 PM + 1200 = 1945 24-hour time

To convert from 24-hour time to traditional time (for times from 1300 to 2400 hours) subtract 12 hours (1200) and insert the colon. For example:

1413 − 1200 = 2:13 PM
1920 − 1200 = 7:20 PM
2345 − 1200 = 11:45 PM

PROBLEMS: THE 24-HOUR CLOCK

Exercise 1

Given the traditional clock time, state the time according to the 24-hour clock.

1. 9 PM _____   6. 10:25 AM _____

2. 4 AM _____   7. 3:30 PM _____

3. 4:05 PM _____   8. 2 AM _____

4. 6:30 AM _____   9. 10 PM _____

5. 8:15 PM _____   10. 12 Midnight _____

Exercise II

Given the time using the 24-hour clock, state the time according to the traditional clock.

1. 1315 hours _____   6. 0230 hours _____

2. 0345 hours _____   7. 0400 hours _____

3. 0620 hours _____   8. 1645 hours _____

4. 2015 hours _____   9. 1010 hours _____

5. 2325 hours _____   10. 2215 hours _____

ANSWERS: THE 24-HOUR CLOCK

Exercise I

1. 9 PM   2100 (or twenty-one hundred) hours

2. 4 AM   0400 (or zero four hundred) hours

3. 4:05 PM   1605 (or sixteen oh five) hours

4. 6:30 AM   0630 (or zero six thirty) hours

5. 8:15 PM   2015 (twenty fifteen) hours

6. 10:25 AM   1025 (or ten twenty-five) hours

7. 3:30 PM   1530 (or fifteen thirty) hours

8. 2 AM   0200 (or zero two hundred) hours

9. 10 PM   2200 (or twenty-two hundred) hours

10. 12 Midnight   2400 (or twenty-four hundred) hours

Exercise II

1. 1315 hours	1:15 PM	6. 0230 hours	2:30 AM
2. 0345 hours	3:45 AM	7. 0400 hours	4:00 AM
3. 0620 hours	6:20 AM	8. 1645 hours	4:45 PM
4. 2015 hours	8:15 PM	9. 1010 hours	10:10 AM
5. 2325 hours	11:25 PM	10. 2215 hours	10:15 PM

Practice Tests

PRACTICE TEST 1

Read all problems carefully. Show all work. Label correctly.

1. Prepare 8 g MgSO₄ for IM administration from a 50% solution.
   Give _____

2. The physician orders aspirin gr viiss. The tablets on hand are gr v tablets.
   Give _____

3. Give Kaon elixir 15 mEq. You have available 20 mEq per 30 ml.
   Give _____

4. Give ampicillin 0.15 g po from a stock bottle labeled 500 mg per 5 ml.
   Give _____

5. Using Clark's rule, determine the child's dose if the adult dose of phenobarbital is 80 mg and the child weighs 45 lb?

6. Prepare 500 ml of 10% glycerin solution from liquid glycerin.
   Drug _____
   Solvent _____

7. Give Keflin 750 mg. Vial is labeled 0.5 g in 2.2 ml. Give _____

8. You have scored tablets of digoxin labeled 0.25 mg. Give 0.000125 g.

9. A drug is labeled gr $\frac{1}{100}$ in ♏ xv. Give gr $\frac{1}{150}$ _____

10. The physician has ordered 1000 ml D_5W to run IV for 8 hours. The drop
    factor is 10 gtt/ml. At what rate should this IV run? _____

11. The physician orders 62 units of NPH insulin to be given before break-
    fast. You have U100 insulin on hand. How would you prepare this dose
    using an insulin syringe?

12. 1 ml   = _____ ♏   1 gtt   = _____ ♏
    ℥ ii   = _____ ℨ   ℨ ii   = _____ ml
    3 Tbs   = _____ oz   15 ml   = _____ tsp
    1 pt   = _____ L   2 pt   = _____ ml
    4000 ml = _____ gal   ℥ iiiss = _____ ml

13. Give 300,000 U of crystalline penicillin IM. In the medicine room you
    find a bottle of 1,000,000 U of crystalline penicillin in dry form. Add 3.6
    ml diluent and shake. Each milliliter contains 500,000 U after reconsti-
    tution. The nurse will give _____

14. Give 750 mg of Prostaphlin IM. In the medicine room you have a 2-g bottle of Prostaphlin. Add 5.7 ml distilled water to the vial. After mixing each 1.5 ml will contain 500 mg. The nurse will give _____

15 & 16. Your patient is going to the O.R. You must give Demerol 60 mg and atropine 0.4 mg IM preoperatively. On hand you have a 2-ml ampule of Demerol containing 50 mg/ml. Give _____ of Demerol. You have atropine 1 mg/cc. Give _____ atropine.

17. Convert the following temperatures.
    104 °F = _____ °C
    35 °C = _____ °F

18. The physician orders gr ⅟₆₀ of a drug. On hand tab gr ⅟₈₀.
    Give _____

19. The physician orders elixir of phenobarbital 6 mg from a stock bottle containing 20 mg per 5 cc. Give _____

20. Prepare 1½ qt of a 1:10 solution of sodium hypochlorite solution.

ANSWERS: PRACTICE TEST 1

1. A 50% solution means that there is 50 gm drug in 100 ml solution; hence in the formula or ratio there is 50 gm of drug per 100 ml of solution.

$$\frac{8\text{ g}}{\cancel{50}\text{ g}} \times \cancel{100}^{2}\text{ ml} = 16\text{ ml MgSO}_4 \qquad 50\text{ g}:100\text{ ml}::8\text{ g}:x\text{ ml}$$

$$\frac{50\text{ g}}{100\text{ ml}} :: \frac{8\text{ g}}{x\text{ ml}}$$

$$50x = 800$$

$$x = 16\text{ ml MgSO}_4$$

2. $\dfrac{7.5 \text{ gr}}{5 \text{ gr}} \times 1 \text{ tab} = \dfrac{7.5}{5}$

$= 1.5 \text{ tab aspirin}$

$5 \text{ gr} : 1 \text{ tab} :: 7\frac{1}{2} \text{ gr} : x \text{ tab}$

$\dfrac{5 \text{ gr}}{1 \text{ tab}} :: \dfrac{7\frac{1}{2} \text{ gr}}{x \text{ tab}}$

$5x = 7\frac{1}{2}$

$x = 1.5 \text{ tab aspirin}$

3. $\dfrac{15 \text{ mEq}}{\underset{2}{\cancel{20} \text{ mEq}}} \times \overset{3}{\cancel{30} \text{ ml}} = \dfrac{45}{2}$

$= 22.5 \text{ ml}$
Kaon elixir

$20 \text{ mEq} : 30 \text{ ml} :: 15 \text{ mEq} : x \text{ ml}$

$\dfrac{20 \text{ mEq}}{30 \text{ ml}} = \dfrac{15 \text{ mEq}}{x \text{ ml}}$

$20x = 450$

$x = 22.5 \text{ ml}$
Kaon elixir

4. $0.15 \text{ g} = 150 \text{ mg}$

$\dfrac{150 \text{ mg}}{\underset{10}{\cancel{500} \text{ mg}}} \times \overset{1}{\cancel{5} \text{ ml}} = \dfrac{15}{10}$

$= 1.5 \text{ ml}$
ampicillin

$500 \text{ mg} : 5 \text{ ml} :: 0.15 \text{ g} : x \text{ ml}$

$\dfrac{500 \text{ mg}}{5 \text{ ml}} = \dfrac{0.15 \text{ g}}{x \text{ ml}}$

$\dfrac{500 \text{ mg}}{5 \text{ ml}} = \dfrac{150 \text{ mg}}{x \text{ ml}}$

$500x = 750$

$x = 1.5 \text{ ml}$
ampicillin

5. $\dfrac{\overset{9}{\cancel{45} \text{ lb}}}{\underset{30}{\cancel{150} \text{ lb}}} \times 80 \text{ mg} = \dfrac{720}{30}$

$= 24 \text{ mg phenobarbital}$

6. $\dfrac{10 \text{ ml}}{\cancel{100} \text{ ml}} \times \overset{5}{\cancel{500}} \text{ ml} = 50 \text{ ml glycerin}$

$\dfrac{10 \text{ ml}}{100 \text{ ml}} = \dfrac{x \text{ ml}}{500 \text{ ml}}$

$100x = 5000$

$x = 50 \text{ ml glycerin}$

$$
\begin{array}{r}
500 \text{ ml solution} \\
- \quad 50 \text{ ml glycerin} \\
\hline
450 \text{ ml solvent}
\end{array}
$$

7. 750 mg = 0.75 g

$\dfrac{0.75 \text{ g}}{0.5 \text{ g}} \times 2.2 \text{ ml} = \dfrac{1.65}{0.5}$

$= 3.3 \text{ ml Keflin}$

$\dfrac{0.5 \text{ g}}{2.2 \text{ ml}} = \dfrac{0.75 \text{ g}}{x \text{ ml}}$

$0.5x = 1.65$

$x = \dfrac{1.65}{0.5}$

$x = 3.3 \text{ ml Keflin}$

8. 0.000125 g = 0.125 mg

$\dfrac{0.125 \text{ mg}}{0.25 \text{ mg}} \times 1 \text{ tab} = \dfrac{0.125}{0.25}$

$= 0.5 \text{ or } \dfrac{1}{2} \text{ tab}$
digoxin

$\dfrac{0.25 \text{ mg}}{1 \text{ tab}} = \dfrac{0.125 \text{ mg}}{x \text{ tab}}$

$0.25x = 0.125$

$x = 0.5 \text{ tab digoxin}$

9. ♏ xv = 15 ♏

$\dfrac{\text{gr } \dfrac{1}{150}}{\text{gr } \dfrac{1}{100}} \times 15 \text{ ♏} = \dfrac{\dfrac{15}{150}}{\dfrac{1}{100}}$

$= \dfrac{15}{150} \div \dfrac{1}{100}$

$= \dfrac{\overset{5}{\cancel{15}}}{\underset{\underset{1}{\cancel{3}}}{\cancel{150}}} \times \dfrac{\overset{2}{\cancel{100}}}{1}$

$= 10 \text{ ♏}$

$\text{gr } \dfrac{1}{100} : 15 \text{ ♏} :: \text{gr } \dfrac{1}{150} : x \text{ ♏}$

$\dfrac{1}{100} x = \dfrac{15}{150}$

$\dfrac{1}{100} x = \dfrac{1}{10}$

$x = \dfrac{1}{10} \div \dfrac{1}{100}$

$x = \dfrac{1}{10} \times \dfrac{100}{1}$

$= \dfrac{100}{10} = 10 \text{ ♏}$

You could also solve this problem by substituting 1 ml for 15 minims:

$$\frac{gr \dfrac{1}{150}}{gr \dfrac{1}{100}} \times 1\ ml = \frac{\dfrac{1}{150}}{\dfrac{1}{100}} = \frac{1}{\cancel{150}\,^{3}} \times \frac{\cancel{100}\,^{2}}{1} = \frac{2}{3} = 0.66\ ml \approx 0.7\ ml$$

10. $1000\ ml \div 8\ hr = 125\ ml/hr\ IV$ to run

$$\frac{Drop\ factor}{Time} \times 1\text{-hr volume} = Flow\ rate$$

$$\frac{\overset{1}{\cancel{10}}\ gtt/ml}{\underset{6}{\cancel{60}}\ min} \times 125\ ml = \frac{125}{6}$$

$$= 20\frac{5}{6} \approx 21\ gtt/min$$

Always round drops to the nearest whole number.

11. Using a U100 syringe draw U100 NPH insulin up to the 62-unit mark on the syringe.

12.

1 ml	=	15	℥	1 gtt	=	1 ℥
℥ II	=	16	ʒ	ʒ ii	=	8 ml
3 Tbs	=	1½	oz	15 ml	=	3 tsp
1 pt	=	0.5	L	2 pt	=	1000 ml
4000 ml	=	1	gal	ʒ iiiss	=	105 ml

13.

$$\frac{\overset{3}{\cancel{300,000}}\ U}{\underset{5}{\cancel{500,000}}\ U} \times 1\ ml = \frac{3}{5}$$

$$= 0.6\ ml$$
crystalline
penicillin

$$\frac{500,000\ U}{1\ ml} :: \frac{300,000\ U}{x\ ml}$$

$$500,000\ x = 300,000$$

$$x = 0.6\ ml$$
crystalline
penicillin

14. $\dfrac{\overset{3}{\cancel{750}}\text{ mg}}{\underset{2}{\cancel{500}}\text{ mg}} \times 1.5 \text{ ml} = \dfrac{4.5}{2}$

$$= 2.25$$
$$\approx 2.3 \text{ ml}$$
$$\text{Prostaphlin}$$

$\dfrac{500 \text{ mg}}{1.5 \text{ ml}} :: \dfrac{750 \text{ mg}}{x \text{ ml}}$

$$500x = 1125$$
$$x = 2.25$$
$$x \approx 2.3 \text{ ml}$$
$$\text{Prostaphlin}$$

15. $\dfrac{6\cancel{0} \text{ mg}}{5\cancel{0} \text{ mg}} \times 1 \text{ ml} = \dfrac{6}{5}$

$$= 1.2 \text{ ml Demerol}$$

$50 \text{ mg} : 1 \text{ ml} :: 60 \text{ mg} : x \text{ ml}$

$\dfrac{50 \text{ mg}}{1 \text{ ml}} :: \dfrac{60 \text{ mg}}{x \text{ ml}}$

$$50x = 60$$
$$x = 1.2 \text{ ml Demerol}$$

16. $\dfrac{0.4 \text{ mg}}{1 \text{ mg}} \times 1 \text{ ml} = 0.4 \text{ ml atropine}$

$1 \text{ mg} : 1 \text{ ml} :: 0.4 \text{ mg} : x \text{ ml}$

$\dfrac{1 \text{ mg}}{1 \text{ ml}} :: \dfrac{0.4 \text{ mg}}{x \text{ ml}}$

$$1x = 0.4$$
$$x = 0.4 \text{ ml atropine}$$

17.

$$1.8 \,^\circ\text{C} = \,^\circ\text{F} - 32$$
$$1.8 \,^\circ\text{C} = 104 - 32$$
$$1.8 \,^\circ\text{C} = 72$$
$$1.8 \div 1.8 \,^\circ\text{C} = 72 \div 1.8$$
$$^\circ\text{C} = 40$$

$$^\circ\text{C} = (^\circ\text{F} - 32) \times \dfrac{5}{9}$$

$$^\circ\text{C} = (104 - 32) \times \dfrac{5}{9}$$

$$^\circ\text{C} = 72 \times \dfrac{5}{9} = \dfrac{360}{9}$$

$$^\circ\text{C} = 40$$

$$1.8 \,^\circ\text{C} = \,^\circ\text{F} - 32$$
$$1.8 \times 35 = \,^\circ\text{F} - 32$$
$$32 + 63 = \,^\circ\text{F} - 32 + 32$$
$$95 = \,^\circ\text{F}$$

$$^\circ\text{F} = \left(\dfrac{9}{5}\,^\circ\text{C}\right) + 32$$

$$^\circ\text{F} = \left(\dfrac{9}{\cancel{5}} \times \overset{7}{\cancel{35}}\right) + 32$$
$$1$$

$$^\circ\text{F} = 63 + 32$$
$$^\circ\text{F} = 95$$

18.

$$\frac{D}{H} \times V = G$$

$$\frac{gr\,\dfrac{1}{60}}{gr\,\dfrac{1}{80}} \times 1 \text{ ml} = \frac{\dfrac{1}{60}}{\dfrac{1}{80}}$$

$$= \frac{1}{\cancel{60}_{3}} \times \frac{\cancel{80}^{4}}{1}$$

$$= \frac{4}{3}$$

$$= 1.33 \approx 1 \text{ tab}$$

$$\frac{gr\,\dfrac{1}{80}}{1 \text{ tab}} :: \frac{gr\,\dfrac{1}{60}}{x \text{ tab}}$$

$$\frac{1}{80x} = \frac{1}{60}$$

$$x = \frac{1}{60} \div \frac{1}{80}$$

$$x = \frac{1}{60} \times \frac{80}{1}$$

$$x = 1.33 \approx 1 \text{ tab}$$

19.

$$\frac{6 \text{ mg}}{\cancel{20} \text{ mg}_{4}} \times \cancel{8}^{1} \text{ ml} = \frac{6}{4}$$

$$= 1.5 \text{ ml}$$

$$20 \text{ mg}:5 \text{ ml}::6 \text{ mg}:x \text{ ml}$$

$$\frac{20 \text{ mg}}{5 \text{ ml}} :: \frac{6 \text{ mg}}{x \text{ ml}}$$

$$20x = 30$$

$$x = 1.5 \text{ ml}$$

20.

$$\frac{1 \text{ ml}}{10 \text{ ml}} \times 1500 \text{ ml} = 150 \text{ ml}$$

$$1 \text{ ml}:10 \text{ ml}::x \text{ ml}:1500 \text{ ml}$$

$$10x = 1500$$

$$x = 150 \text{ ml}$$

$$\begin{array}{r} 1500 \text{ ml solution} \\ - \ \ 150 \text{ ml solute} \\ \hline 1350 \text{ ml solvent} \end{array}$$

PRACTICE TEST 2

1. The physician orders 7500 U of heparin SC every 12 hours. Calculate the amount of heparin solution necessary to administer 7500 U heparin per dose. Shade the syringe to the correct dose.

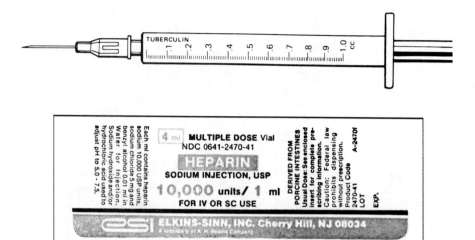

2. A child under 9 years of age should receive 1 mg/kg aminophylline per hour.

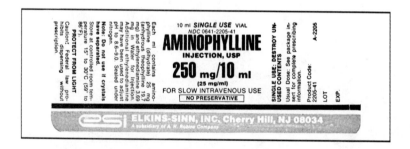

a. How much aminophylline should a 44-lb child receive?

b. How much aminophylline solution is necessary to administer the recommended dosage?

3. The nurse is to add the 20 mg aminophylline in problem 2 to a Buretrol. The child is to receive 50 ml IV fluid per hour. How much IV fluid should be added to the Buretrol? If the drop factor is 60 gtt/ml, what flow rate should be used?

4. The physician orders 0.32 mg of atropine. You have atropine sulfate for injection. How much solution is to be given sc? Mark the syringe to the correct calibration.

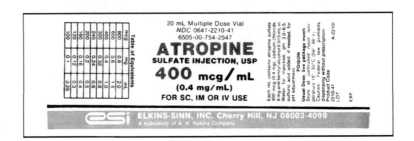

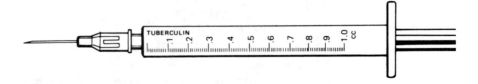

5. Add 2 g lidocaine to 250 ml IV solution. How much lidocaine solution should be added? You have a 2 percent lidocaine solution.

6. You need to administer 4 mg lidocaine per minute using the IV solution mixed in problem 5. You have 2 g lidocaine in 250 ml solution. How many milliliters of solution should be infused per minute?
   What would be the flow rate if the drop factor is 60 gtt/ml?
   What would be the flow rate if the drop factor is 20 gtt/ml?

7. Mrs. Block is to receive 500 mg of calcium gluconate IV push over 10 minutes. How much solution should be administered?

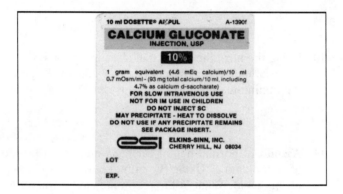

8. The physician orders atropine 0.05 mg for an infant preoperatively. How much solution should be given? Mark the syringe shown below to the correct calibration.

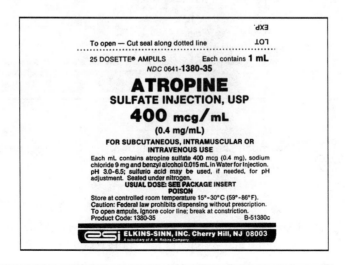

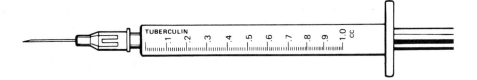

9. If the recommended dosage range of atropine for a child is 0.01 to 0.4 mg/kg/dose, what is the dosage range of atropine for a child who weighs 6.4 kg?

10. Using the atropine drug label shown in problem 8, and using the dosage range obtained for the child who weighs 6.4 kg in problem 9, calculate the minimum and maximum dosage that may be administered.

11. A child of normal height for his weight (15 lb) is to receive 0.2 mg/m^2 of scopolamine. Using the nomogram on page 247, determine the BSA of this child. What is the recommended dosage for this child?

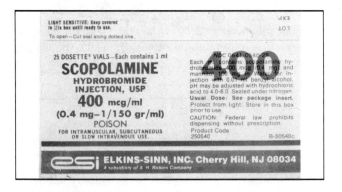

12. How much scopolamine solution should be administered to the child in problem 11?

13. Using the nomogram on page 247, determine the BSA of a child who is 90 cm tall and weighs 19 kg? If the recommended dosage of scopolamine

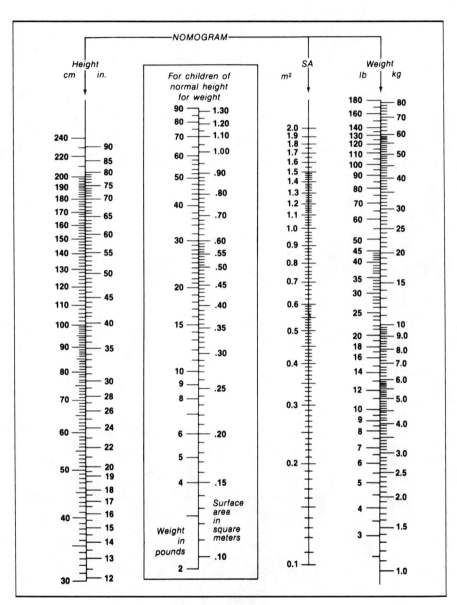

Nomogram for use with problems 11 and 13.

is 0.2 mg/m², how many milligrams of scopolamine should the child receive?

14. How much scopolamine solution should be administered to the child in problem 13? Shade in the syringe pictured below to the correct level. (Refer to the label shown in problem 11.)

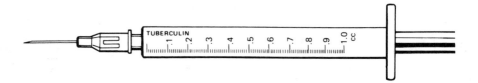

15. The physician orders scopolamine gr ½₀₀ sc stat. How much solution should be given? (Refer to the label shown in problem 11.) Shade the syringe shown below to the proper level.

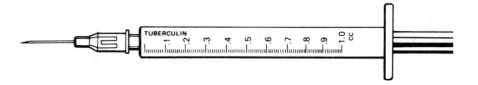

16. The physician orders cyanocobalamin (vitamine B₁₂) 100 mcg/day sc for 5 days. (See label below.) How much cyanocobalamin solution should be given? Shade the syringe shown below to the proper level.

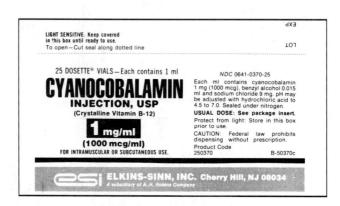

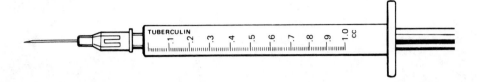

17. The physician order states: Add 10 g MgSO₄ (magnesium sulfate) to 1000 ml D₅W (5% dextrose in water). Administer 1.5 g/hr.

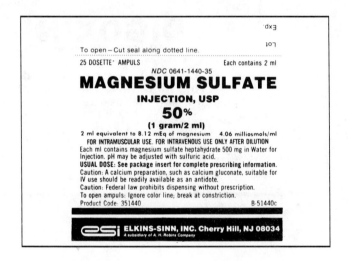

a. How much magnesium sulfate solution should be added to the 1000 ml D₅W?

b. How much IV solution will be needed to administer 1.5 g/hr?

c. Administer the IV using an IV administration set with a drop factor of 20 gtt/ml.

d. Administer the IV using an IV administration set with a drop factor of 60 gtt/ml.

18. The physician orders 1 mg digoxin as a loading dose. How much solution should be administered?

To open, cut seal along dotted line.   10⁊

100 DOSETTE* AMPULS   Each contains 2 ml

NDC 0641-1410-36

DIGOXIN
INJECTION, USP

500 mcg /2 ml
(0.5 mg/2 ml—250 mcg/ml)
FOR SLOW INTRAVENOUS OR DEEP INTRAMUSCULAR USE.
DILUTION IS NOT REQUIRED

Each ml contains digoxin 250 mcg (0.25 mg), alcohol 0.1 ml, propylene glycol 0.4 ml, dibasic sodium phosphate anhydrous 3 mg and citric acid anhydrous 0.8 mg in Water for Injection. pH 6.7-7.3 (additional citric acid and/or sodium phosphate added, if necessary, for pH adjustment). Sealed under nitrogen.
STORE AT CONTROLLED ROOM TEMPERATURE 15° TO 30°C (59° TO 86°F).
USUAL DOSE: See package insert.
Caution: Federal law prohibits dispensing without prescription.
To open ampuls, ignore color line; break at constriction.
Product Code 1410-36   B-61410e

ELKINS-SINN, INC. Cherry Hill, NJ 08034
A subsidiary of A. H. Robins Company

19. The loading dose of digoxin for a premature infant is 0.04 mg/kg IV divided into three doses over 24 hours. (Refer to the digoxin label in problem 18.)
    a. How much digoxin should a premature infant weighing 3 kg receive?

    b. How much digoxin solution is necessary in order to administer this dose?

20. The physician orders 40 mg gentamicin to be given IM. How much gentamicin solution should be administered?

25 DOSETTE® SYRINGES
(5 trays of 5 each)

Each contains **1.5** ml

NDC 0641-6308-15

GENTAMICIN

SULFATE INJECTION, USP

60 mg/1.5 ml*

(40 mg/ml)

FOR INTRAVENOUS OR INTRAMUSCULAR USE. DILUTE BEFORE USING INTRAVENOUSLY.

Each ml contains *gentamicin sulfate equivalent to gentamicin 40 mg in Water for Injection with 1.8 mg methylparaben, 0.2 mg propylparaben, 0.1 mg edetate disodium and 3.2 mg sodium bisulfite. Sodium hydroxide is used to adjust pH to 3.0–5.5; sulfuric acid used, if needed. Sealed under nitrogen.

USUAL ADULT DOSE: See package insert for complete prescribing information.

Caution: Federal law prohibits dispensing without prescription.

DO NOT USE IF PRECIPITATED

22 gauge, 1¼″ needle

STORE AT CONTROLLED
ROOM TEMPERATURE
15°-30°C (59°-86°F)
AVOID FREEZING

Product Code 6308-15

B-56308

To open—Cut along dotted line—Pull out end flap

ΘSi ELKINS-SINN, INC. Cherry Hill, NJ 08034
A subsidiary of A. H. Robins Company

ANSWERS: PRACTICE TEST 2

1. $\dfrac{7500 \text{ U}}{10{,}000 \text{ U}} \times 1 \text{ ml} = \dfrac{75}{100}$

   $= 0.75 \text{ ml}$
   heparin
   solution

   $10{,}000 \text{ U} : 1 \text{ ml} :: 7500 \text{ U} : x \text{ ml}$

   $10{,}000x = 7500$

   $x = 0.75 \text{ ml}$
   heparin
   solution

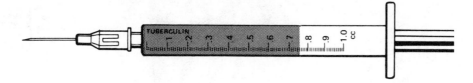

2. First convert 44 lb to kilograms:

$$44 \text{ lb} \div 2.2 = 20 \text{ kg}$$

a. The dose for a child under 9 years of age is 1 mg/kg/hr. A 20-kg child should receive

$$1 \text{ mg/kg/hr} \times 20 \text{ kg} = 20 \text{ mg/hr}$$

b. $\dfrac{20 \text{ mg}}{25 \text{ mg}} \times 1 \text{ ml} = \dfrac{4}{5}$ $\dfrac{25 \text{ mg}}{1 \text{ ml}} :: \dfrac{20 \text{ mg}}{x \text{ ml}}$

$$= 0.8 \text{ ml}$$ $25x = 20$
aminophylline
solution $x = 0.8 \text{ ml}$
                            aminophylline
                            solution

3. Add approximately 25 ml of the needed amount of IV solution to the buretrol then add 0.8 ml aminophylline. Shake to mix and then fill the buretrol to the 50-ml level. Mix thoroughly.

50 ml IV/hr $\dfrac{60 \text{ gtt/ml}}{60 \text{ min}} \times 50 \text{ ml} = 50 \text{ gtt/min}$
-0.8 ml aminophylline
$\overline{49.2 \text{ ml of IV fluid}}$ IV flow rate

4. 0.32 mg = 320 mcg

$$\dfrac{\overset{4}{\cancel{320}} \text{ mcg}}{\underset{5}{\cancel{400}} \text{ mcg}} \times 1 \text{ ml} = \dfrac{4}{5}$$ $400 \text{ mcg} : 1 \text{ ml} :: 320 \text{ mcg} : x \text{ ml}$

$400x = 320$

$$= 0.8 \text{ ml}$$ $x = \dfrac{320}{400}$
atropine
                            $x = 0.8 \text{ ml}$
                            atropine

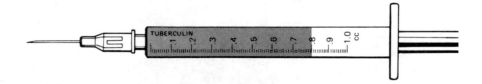

Read the label to check your answer. This label states the equivalents and dose.

5. A 2% solution contains 2 g drug in every 100 ml solution or 20 mg/ml.

$$2 \text{ g} = 2000 \text{ mg}$$

$$\frac{2 \text{ g}}{100 \text{ ml}} = 2\% \text{ solution}$$

$$\frac{\overset{100}{\cancel{2000} \text{ mg}}}{\underset{1}{\cancel{20} \text{ mg}}} \times 1 \text{ ml} = 100 \text{ ml}$$
lidocaine
solution

$$\frac{20 \text{ mg}}{1 \text{ ml}} :: \frac{2000 \text{ mg}}{x \text{ ml}}$$

$$20x = 2000$$

$$x = 100 \text{ ml}$$
lidocaine
solution

Two vials of 2% lidocaine are needed: each one contains 50 ml.

6. $\dfrac{4 \text{ mg}}{\underset{40}{\cancel{2000} \text{ mg}}} \times \overset{5}{\cancel{250}} \text{ ml} = \dfrac{20}{40}$

$$\frac{2000 \text{ mg}}{250 \text{ ml}} :: \frac{4 \text{ mg}}{x \text{ ml}}$$

$$= \frac{1}{2} = 0.5 \text{ ml}$$
lidocaine

$$2000x = 1000$$

$$x = 0.5 \text{ ml}$$
lidocaine
solution

IV Formula:

$$\frac{\text{DF}}{\text{Time}} \times \text{volume} = \text{gtt/min}$$

$$\frac{60 \text{ gtt/ml}}{1 \text{ min}} \times 0.5 \text{ ml} = 30 \text{ gtt/min}$$
IV flow rate

$$\frac{20 \text{ gtt/ml}}{1 \text{ min}} \times 0.5 \text{ ml} = 10 \text{ gtt/min}$$
IV flow rate

7. A 10% solution contains 10 g calcium per 100 ml solution or 1 g per 10 ml.

$$1 \text{ g} = 1000 \text{ mg}$$

$$\frac{\overset{1}{\cancel{500} \text{ mg}}}{\underset{2}{\cancel{1000} \text{ mg}}} \times 10 \text{ ml} = \frac{10}{2}$$

$$\frac{1000 \text{ mg}}{10 \text{ ml}} :: \frac{500 \text{ mg}}{x \text{ ml}}$$

$$= 5 \text{ ml}$$
calcium
gluconate

$$1000x = 5000$$

$$x = 5 \text{ ml}$$
calcium
gluconate

Note: 4.6 mEq calcium is the amount of elemental calcium in the solution. This is not used in solving the problem.

8. 0.05 mg = 50 mcg

$$\frac{\overset{1}{\cancel{50}\,\text{mcg}}}{\underset{8}{\cancel{400}\,\text{mcg}}} \times 1\ \text{ml} = 0.125$$

$$\approx 0.13\ \text{ml}$$
atropine sulfate

$$\frac{400\ \text{mcg}}{1\ \text{ml}} :: \frac{50\ \text{mcg}}{x\ \text{ml}}$$

$$400x = 50$$

$$x = 0.125$$

$$\approx 0.13\ \text{ml}$$
atropine sulfate

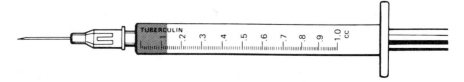

9.   0.01 mg/kg = child's minimum dose of atropine

0.01 mg/kg × 6.4 kg = 0.064 mg ≈ 0.06 mg

0.4 mg/kg = child's maximum dose of atropine

0.4 mg/kg × 6.4 kg = 2.56 mg

10. 0.06 mg = 60 mcg = minimum dose

$$\frac{60\ \text{mcg}}{400\ \text{mcg}} \times 1\ \text{ml} = 0.15\ \text{ml}$$
atropine

$$\frac{400\ \text{mcg}}{1\ \text{ml}} :: \frac{60\ \text{mcg}}{x\ \text{ml}}$$

$$400x = 60$$

$$x = 0.15\ \text{ml atropine}$$

2.56 mg = 2560 mcg = maximum dose

$$\frac{2560\ \text{mcg}}{400\ \text{mcg}} \times 1\ \text{ml} = 6.4\ \text{ml}$$
atropine

$$\frac{400\ \text{mcg}}{1\ \text{ml}} :: \frac{2560\ \text{mcg}}{x\ \text{ml}}$$

$$400x = 2560$$

$$x = 6.4\ \text{ml atropine}$$

It would be better to use a more concentrated strength of atropine for the maximum dose.

11. a. The child's BSA is 0.36 m².

    b. 0.2 mg/m² × 0.36 m² = 0.072 mg = 72 mcg

12. $\dfrac{72 \text{ mcg}}{400 \text{ mcg}} \times 1 \text{ ml} = \dfrac{72}{400}$

$$= 0.18 \text{ ml}$$
scopolamine

$\dfrac{400 \text{ mcg}}{1 \text{ ml}} :: \dfrac{72 \text{ mcg}}{x \text{ ml}}$

$400x = 72$

$x = 0.18 \text{ ml}$
scopolamine

13. a. A child of 90 cm height and 19 kg weight has a BSA of 0.7 m².

    b. 0.2 mg/m² × 0.7 m² = 0.14 mg scopolamine

14. 0.14 mg = 140 mcg

$\dfrac{140 \text{ mcg}}{400 \text{ mcg}} \times 1 \text{ ml} = 0.35 \text{ ml}$
scopolamine

$\dfrac{400 \text{ mcg}}{1 \text{ ml}} :: \dfrac{140 \text{ mcg}}{x \text{ ml}}$

$400x = 140$

$x = 0.35 \text{ ml scopolamine}$

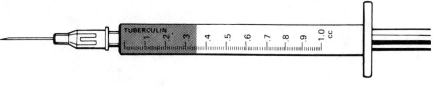

15. $\dfrac{\text{gr } \dfrac{1}{200}}{\text{gr } \dfrac{1}{150}} \times 1 \text{ ml} = \dfrac{\dfrac{1}{200}}{\dfrac{1}{150}}$

$$= \dfrac{1}{200} \div \dfrac{1}{150}$$

$$= \dfrac{1}{\cancel{200}} \times \dfrac{\cancel{150}^{\,3}}{1}$$

$$= \dfrac{3}{4}$$

$$= 0.75 \text{ ml}$$
scopolamine

$\dfrac{\text{gr } \dfrac{1}{150}}{1 \text{ ml}} :: \dfrac{\text{gr } \dfrac{1}{200}}{x \text{ ml}}$

$\dfrac{1}{150x} = \dfrac{1}{200}$

$x = \dfrac{1}{200} \div \dfrac{1}{150}$

$x = \dfrac{1}{\cancel{200}} \times \dfrac{\cancel{150}^{\,3}}{1}$

$x = \dfrac{3}{4}$

$$= 0.75 \text{ ml}$$
scopolamine

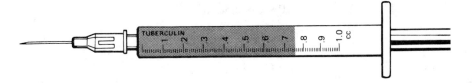

16.
$$\frac{\overset{1}{\cancel{100}\text{ mcg}}}{\underset{10}{\cancel{1000}\text{ mcg}}} \times 1\text{ ml} = 0.1\text{ ml}$$
cyano-
cobalamin

$$\frac{1000\text{ mcg}}{1\text{ ml}} :: \frac{100\text{ mcg}}{x\text{ ml}}$$

$$1000x = 100$$

$$x = 0.1\text{ ml}$$
cyano-
cobalamin

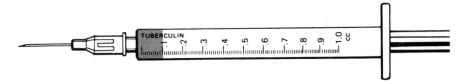

17.
a. $\dfrac{10\text{ g}}{1\text{ g}} \times 2\text{ ml} = 20\text{ ml}$
MgSO$_4$ solution

$$\frac{1\text{ g}}{2\text{ ml}} :: \frac{10\text{ g}}{x\text{ ml}}$$

$$1x = 20$$

$$x = 20\text{ ml MgSO}_4\text{ solution}$$

You would add the contents of 10 ampules to the IV.

b. $\dfrac{1.5\text{ g}}{\underset{1}{\cancel{10}\text{ g}}} \times \overset{100}{\cancel{1000}}\text{ ml} = 150\text{ ml MgSO}_4\text{ solution per hour}$

c. $\dfrac{\underset{3}{\cancel{20}\text{ gtt/ml}}}{\cancel{60}\text{ min}} \times \overset{50}{\cancel{150}}\text{ ml} = 50\text{ gtt/min}$
       1

d. $\dfrac{\overset{1}{\cancel{60}\text{ gtt/ml}}}{\underset{1}{\cancel{60}\text{ min}}} \times 150\text{ ml} = 150\text{ gtt/min}$

18. $\dfrac{1\ \text{mg}}{0.5\ \text{mg}} \times 2\ \text{ml} = \dfrac{2}{0.5}$

$= 4\ \text{ml digoxin}$

$\dfrac{0.5\ \text{mg}}{2\ \text{ml}} :: \dfrac{1\ \text{mg}}{x\ \text{ml}}$

$0.5x = 2$

$x = 4\ \text{ml digoxin}$

19. a. $0.04\ \text{mg/kg} \times 3\ \text{kg} = 0.12\ \text{mg per day} \div 3\ \text{doses} = 0.04\ \text{mg/dose}$

 b. $0.04\ \text{mg} = 40\ \text{mcg}$

$\dfrac{40\ \text{mcg}}{500\ \text{mcg}} \times 2\ \text{ml} = \dfrac{8}{50}$

$= 0.16\ \text{ml digoxin}$

$\dfrac{500\ \text{mcg}}{2\ \text{ml}} :: \dfrac{40\ \text{mcg}}{x\ \text{ml}}$

$500x = 80$

$x = 0.16\ \text{ml digoxin}$

OR

$\dfrac{0.04\ \text{mg}}{0.5\ \text{mg}} \times 2\ \text{ml} = \dfrac{0.08}{0.5}$

$= 0.16\ \text{ml digoxin}$

20. $\dfrac{\overset{2}{\cancel{40}}\ \text{mg}}{\underset{3}{\cancel{60}}\ \text{mg}} \times 1.5\ \text{ml} = \dfrac{3.0}{3}$

$= 1\ \text{ml}$
gentamicin

$\dfrac{60\ \text{mg}}{1.5\ \text{ml}} :: \dfrac{40\ \text{mg}}{x\ \text{ml}}$

$60x = 60$

$x = 1\ \text{ml gentamicin}$

PRACTICE TEST 3

Read and solve all problems carefully. Accuracy is important. Label your answers correctly. SHOW YOUR WORK.

1. 5 gr	=	_____ g	0400	=	_____	Traditional time
3 kg	=	_____ lb	1:10 PM	=	_____	24-hour clock
1 ml	=	_____ ♏	2 ℥	=	_____	℈
1.5 L	=	_____ pt	4 tsp	=	_____	℥
6 T	=	_____ oz	3 gal	=	_____	qt

2. The physician orders sodium bicarbonate 0.64 g. The sodium bicarbonate on hand is available in 320-mg capsules. Give _____

3. The physician orders aspirin gr xx. The aspirin on hand is available in gr v tablets. Give _____

4. The physician ordered Dilantin 100 mg for Mr. Smith. You have Dilantin 125 mg per 5 ml. Give _____

5. The physician has ordered 200 ml of an IV drug to be given in 45 minutes. The drop factor is 10 gtt/cc. At what rate should this IV run? _____

6. Prepare 1000 ml of 10 percent solution from a 30 percent solution. Amount of solute _____ Amount of solvent _____

7. The physician orders 60 mg of Thorazine. It is available in a vial containing 0.025 g/ml. Give _____

8. Mr. Brown is to receive 30 mg/kg/day of a drug. How much drug should he receive per day if he weighs 176 lb? If the medication is to be given in four equal doses, how much drug should he be given per dose?

Convert the following temperatures:

9. 102 °F = _____ °C

10. 35 °C = _____ °F

11. The physician orders 56 units of PZI insulin. You have U100 PZI insulin.

State how you would prepare this medication. *Shade* the correct syringe to the correct dosage.

_____
_____
_____

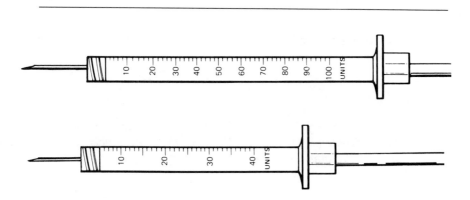

Solve this problem so that you are able to administer the insulin in a tuberculin syringe. Shade the syringe to the correct dose.

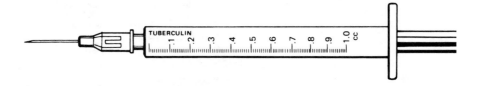

12. The physician orders atropine gr ½₀₀. You have gr ¹⁄₁₀₀ tablets. Give _____

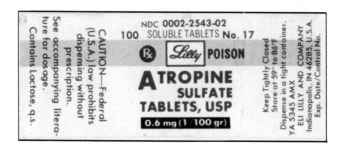

13. You are asked to administer 125 mEq of a drug. The drug available is labeled 75 mEq per 1.5 ml. Give _____

14. You are asked to administer liver extract 160 mcg. The available liver extract is labeled 0.2 mg per 1.5 ml. Give _____

Solve problems 15 through 18 using the drug labels. Read the label and answer the questions about the label.

15.

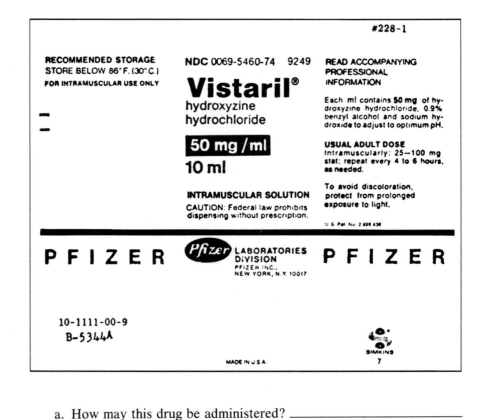

a. How may this drug be administered? _____

b. What is the generic name of this drug? _____

c. If the physician orders 75 mg of Vistaril, how much solution will you administer? _____

16.

a. What type of drug preparation is this? _____

b. List the four special instructions for this drug.
   (1) _____
   (2) _____
   (3) _____
   (4) _____

c. Using the drug manufacturer's recommendation, what is the recommended dose for a child weighing 32 kg? _____
   Explain your answer.

d. How many milliliters of Dynapen will be needed to administer 100 mg of drug?

17. Administer 0.75 g ampicillin.

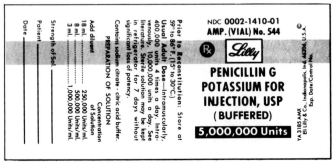

BRISTOL® NDC 0015-7404-20
6505-00-993-3518

Polycillin-N®

STERILE AMPICILLIN
SODIUM For I.M. or I.V. Use
EQUIVALENT TO

1 gram AMPICILLIN

CAUTION: Federal law prohibits
dispensing without prescription.

BRISTOL LABORATORIES
Div. of Bristol-Myers Company
Syracuse, New York 13201

For I.M. use, add 3.5 ml diluent (read
accompanying circular). Resulting solution contains 250 mg ampicillin per ml.

Use solution within 1 hour.

This vial contains ampicillin sodium
equivalent to 1 gm ampicillin.

Usual Dosage:
Adults—250 to 500 mg I.M. q. 6H.

READ ACCOMPANYING CIRCULAR
for detailed indications, I.M. or I.V.
dosage and precautions.

740420DRL-14

© 1977 Bristol Laboratories

Lot
Exp. Date

a. How would you prepare this drug? _____

_____

b. How much solution will you give? _____

18. Physician's order: Potassium penicillin 300,000 U qid.

NDC 0002-1410-01
AMP. (VIAL) No. 544

℞ *Lilly*

PENICILLIN G
POTASSIUM FOR
INJECTION, USP
(BUFFERED)
5,000,000 Units

Prior to Reconstitution: Store at
59° to 86° F. (15° to 30°C).
Usual **Adult Dose**—Intramuscularly,
400,000 units 4 times a day. Intravenously, 10,000,000 units a day. See
literature. Sterile solution may be kept
in refrigerator for 7 days without
significant loss of potency.
Contains sodium citrate · citric acid buffer.

PREPARATION OF SOLUTION

Add diluent	Concentration of Solution
18 ml.	250,000 Units/ml.
8 ml.	500,000 Units/ml.
3 ml.	1,000,000 Units/ml.

Strength of Sol. _____
Patient _____
Date _____

YA 3185 AMX
Eli Lilly & Co., Indianapolis, Ind. 46206, U.S.A.
Exp. Date/Control No.

a. How much diluent must you add to make the strength
   needed? _____

b. What is the dosage strength of the solution you mixed? _____

c. How much potassium penicillin G does this vial contain? _____

d. How much solution must be given to administer 300,000 U? _____

Problems 19 through 21 apply to the following:

Gregory, a 7-month-old infant with H influenza meningitis is to receive an infusion of 150 mg ampicillin in 100 ml D$_5$W via a Buretrol given slowly over a 4-hour period. You have a 500-mg vial. The mixing instructions on the ampicillin vial state: add 1.8 ml diluent. The resulting solution contains 250 mg/ml.

19. a. How would you reconstitute this vial of ampicillin?

    b. How many milliliters of ampicillin should be added to the Buretrol? _____ How much D$_5$W? _____

20. At how many drops per minute should this IV be set if the drop factor is 60 gtt/ml?

21. Gregory's IV was hung at 1200. At 1500 there was 30 ml left. Is this IV on time? If not, recalculate the infusion rate.

Questions 22 and 23 are related.

22. Jane, a 6-month-old infant weighing 10.2 lb, is to receive 4 mg of amphotericin B in 9 ml sterile water for injection added to 40 ml of D$_5$W. You are to administer over a 4-hour period. If the drop factor is 15 gtt/ml, what should the flow rate be? _____ If the drop factor is 60 gtt/ml, what should the flow rate be? _____

23. If the manufacturer of amphotericin states the child's dose of amphotericin is 0.25 to 1 mg/kg/day, is 4 mg an appropriate dose for Jane?

Questions 24 and 25 are related.

24. The physician orders 12.5 mg of drug A to be placed in 50 ml of sodium chloride for injection to be administered over 30 minutes q8h to Amanda, using a microdrip administration set with a drop factor of 60 gtt/ml. What flow rate should be used?

25. Amanda is a 7-month-old infant weighing 13 lb 4 oz. The safe recommended dose of drug A for infants over 7 days of age is 7.5 mg/kg/day in three equal doses. Is the amount ordered by the doctor appropriate for Amanda?

26. Mr. Heart is to receive lidocaine 2 percent solution by IV infusion. The recommended amount is 0.025 ml/kg/min.

    a. How much lidocaine should Mr. Heart receive? He weighs 143 lb.

    b. If the drop factor is 60 gtt/ml, how fast should this IV infuse?

    c. If the drop factor is 20 gtt/ml, how fast should this IV infuse?

27. Using the West nomogram on page 265, determine the BSA (m^2) for a child of normal height and weight if the child's weight is:

    a. 11 lb   = _____ m^2

    b. 26 lb   = _____ m^2

    c. 62.5 lb = _____ m^2

    d. 4 lb   = _____ m^2

    e. 15 lb   = _____ m^2

28. What is the BSA using the West nomogram on page 265 for the following children?

Height	Weight	BSA
a. 110 cm	25 kg	_____ m^2

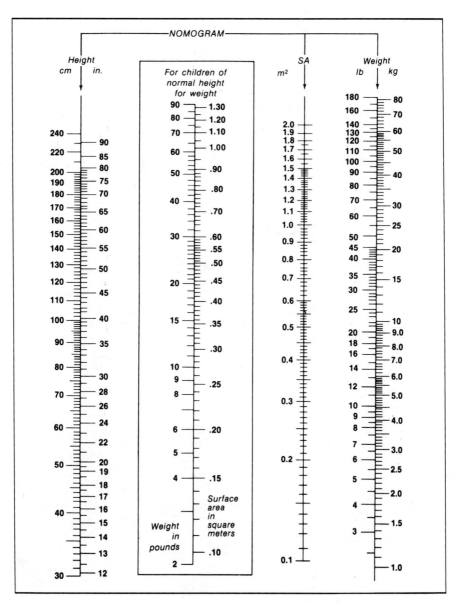

Nomogram for use with problems 27 and 28 of practice test 3, and problem 25 of practice test 4.

Height	Weight	BSA
b. 64 cm	8.2 kg	_____ m^2
c. 19 in	7 lb	_____ m^2
d. 26 in	18.5 lb	_____ m^2
e. 85 cm	19 kg	_____ m^2

29. If the BSA for a child is 0.22 m^2, what is the dose for drug C if the adult dose is 75 mg/dose?

30. What is the recommended dose of Cytoxan for a 10-year-old child with a BSA of 1.2 m^2 if the recommended dosage range is 60 to 250 mg/m^2?

ANSWERS: PRACTICE TEST 3

1. 5 gr = __0.3__ g   0400 = __4:00__ AM traditional time

   3 kg = __6.6__ lb   1:10 PM = __1310__ 24-hour clock

   1 ml = __15 or 16__ m   2 ℥ = __16__ ℨ

   1.5 L = __3__ pt   4 tsp = __4__ ℨ

   6 T = __3__ oz   3 gal = __12__ qt

2. 0.64 g = 640 mg

$$\frac{\overset{2}{\cancel{640}\text{ mg}}}{\underset{1}{\cancel{320}\text{ mg}}} \times 1 \text{ cap} = 2 \text{ cap}$$

$$\frac{320 \text{ mg}}{1 \text{ cap}} :: \frac{640 \text{ mg}}{x \text{ cap}}$$

$$320x = 640$$
$$x = 2 \text{ cap}$$

Give 2 capsules of sodium bicarbonate.

3. gr x = 20 gr   gr v = 5 gr

$$\frac{\overset{4}{\cancel{20}\text{ gr}}}{\underset{1}{\cancel{5}\text{ gr}}} \times 1 \text{ tab} = 4 \text{ tab}$$

$$\frac{5 \text{ gr}}{1 \text{ tab}} :: \frac{20 \text{ gr}}{x \text{ tab}}$$

$$5x = 20$$
$$x = 4 \text{ tab}$$

Give 4 tablets of aspirin.

4.
$$\frac{\overset{4}{\cancel{100 \text{ mg}}}}{\underset{\cancel{5}}{\cancel{125 \text{ mg}}}} \times \overset{1}{\cancel{5}} \text{ ml} = 4 \text{ ml}$$
$$1$$

$$\frac{125 \text{ mg}}{5 \text{ ml}} :: \frac{100 \text{ mg}}{x \text{ ml}}$$
$$125x = 500$$
$$x = 4 \text{ ml}$$

Give 4 ml of Dilantin.

5.
$$\frac{10 \text{ gtt/ml}}{\underset{9}{\cancel{45} \text{ min}}} \times \overset{40}{\cancel{200}} \text{ ml} = \frac{400}{9}$$

$$= 44.4 \approx 44 \text{ gtt/min}$$

6.
$$\frac{\overset{1}{\cancel{10 \text{ ml}}}}{\underset{3}{\cancel{30 \text{ ml}}}} \times 1000 \text{ ml} = \frac{1000}{3}$$

$$\frac{10 \text{ ml}}{30 \text{ ml}} :: \frac{x \text{ ml}}{1000 \text{ ml}}$$
$$30x = 10,000$$
$$x = 333.3 \text{ ml}$$

$$= 333.3 \text{ ml}$$

$$1000.0 \text{ ml solution}$$
$$\underline{-333.3 \text{ ml solute}}$$
$$666.7 \text{ ml solvent}$$

7. 60 mg = 0.06 g

$$\frac{0.06 \text{ g}}{0.025 \text{ g}} \times 1 \text{ ml} = 2.4 \text{ ml}$$

$$\frac{0.025 \text{ g}}{1 \text{ ml}} :: \frac{0.06 \text{ g}}{x \text{ ml}}$$
$$0.025x = 0.06$$
$$x = 2.4 \text{ ml}$$

Give 2.4 ml Thorazine.

8. 176 lb ÷ 2.2 lb/kg = 80 kg

$$30 \text{ mg/kg/day} \times 80 \text{ kg} = 2400 \text{ mg/day}$$
$$2400 \text{ mg} \div 4 \text{ doses} = 600 \text{ mg/dose}$$

9. $1.8 \text{ °C} = \text{°F} - 32$

$1.8 \text{ °C} = 102 - 32$

$\dfrac{1.8 \text{ °C}}{1.8} = \dfrac{70}{1.8}$

$\text{°C} = 38.88 \approx 38.9°$

$\text{°C} = (\text{°F} - 32) \times \dfrac{5}{9}$

$\text{°C} = (102 - 32) \times \dfrac{5}{9}$

$\text{°C} = 70 \times \dfrac{5}{9}$

$\text{°C} = \dfrac{350}{9} \approx 38.88$

$\text{°C} \approx 38.9°$

10. $1.8 \text{ °C} = \text{°F} - 32$

$1.8 \times 35 = \text{°F} - 32$

$32 + 63 = \text{°F} - 32 + 32$

$95 = \text{°F}$

$\text{°F} = \left(\dfrac{9}{5} \text{ C}\right) + 32$

$\text{°F} = \left(\dfrac{9}{5} \times 35°\right) + 32$

$\text{°F} = \left(\dfrac{315}{5}\right) + 32$

$\text{°F} = 63. + 32$

$\text{°F} = 95$

11. Use a U100 syringe.

Draw U100 PZ1 insulin up to 56-unit mark of the U100 insulin syringe:

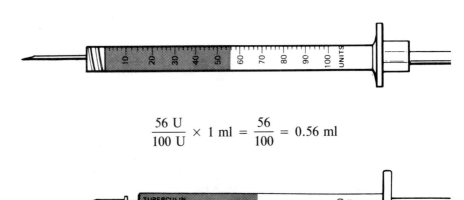

$$\dfrac{56 \text{ U}}{100 \text{ U}} \times 1 \text{ ml} = \dfrac{56}{100} = 0.56 \text{ ml}$$

12.

$$\dfrac{\text{gr } \dfrac{1}{200}}{\text{gr } \dfrac{1}{100}} \times 1 \text{ tab} = \dfrac{\dfrac{1}{200}}{\dfrac{1}{100}}$$

$$= \dfrac{1}{\underset{2}{\cancel{200}}} \times \dfrac{\cancel{100}}{1}$$

$$= \dfrac{1}{2} \text{ tab}$$

$$\dfrac{\text{gr } \dfrac{1}{100}}{1 \text{ tab}} :: \dfrac{\dfrac{1}{200}}{x \text{ tab}}$$

$$\dfrac{1}{100} x = \dfrac{1}{200}$$

$$x = \dfrac{1}{\underset{2}{\cancel{200}}} \times \dfrac{\cancel{100}}{1}$$

$$x = \dfrac{1}{2} \text{ tab}$$

Give ½ tablet of atropine.

13.

$$\dfrac{\overset{5}{\cancel{125}} \text{ mEq}}{\underset{\underset{1}{\cancel{3}}}{\cancel{75} \text{ mEq}}} \times \overset{0.5}{\cancel{1.5}} \text{ ml} = 2.5 \text{ ml}$$

$$\dfrac{75 \text{ mEq}}{1.5 \text{ ml}} :: \dfrac{125 \text{ mEq}}{x \text{ ml}}$$

$$75x = 187.5$$

$$x = 2.5 \text{ ml}$$

Give 2.5 ml of drug.

14. 160 mcg = 0.16 mg

$$\dfrac{\overset{0.8}{\cancel{0.16} \text{ mg}}}{\underset{1}{\cancel{0.2} \text{ mg}}} \times 1.5 \text{ ml} = 1.2 \text{ ml}$$

$$\dfrac{0.2 \text{ mg}}{1.5 \text{ ml}} :: \dfrac{0.16}{x \text{ ml}}$$

$$0.2x = 0.24$$

$$x = 1.2 \text{ ml}$$

Give 1.2 ml liver extract.

15. a. Intramuscularly

b. Hydroxyzine hydrochloride

c.

$$\dfrac{\overset{3}{\cancel{75} \text{ mg}}}{\underset{2}{\cancel{50} \text{ mg}}} \times 1 \text{ ml} = \dfrac{3}{2}$$

$$= 1.5 \text{ ml}$$

$$\dfrac{50 \text{ mg}}{1 \text{ ml}} :: \dfrac{75 \text{ mg}}{x \text{ ml}}$$

$$50x = 75$$

$$x = 1.5 \text{ ml}$$

Give 1.5 ml Vistaril.

16. a. Oral suspension

    b. (1) Store in refrigerator; discard after 14 days.
       (2) Keep bottle tightly closed.
       (3) Shake well before using.
       (4) Federal law prohibits dispensing without a prescription.

    c. 12.5 mg/kg × 32 kg = 400 mg/day ÷ 4

    = 100 mg/dose

The prescribed dose and recommended dose are the same.

d.
$$\frac{\overset{12.5}{\cancel{100\ mg}}}{\cancel{62.5\ mg}} \times \overset{1}{\cancel{5}}\ ml = \frac{100}{12.5}$$

$$= 8\ ml$$

$$\frac{62.5\ mg}{5\ ml} :: \frac{100\ mg}{x\ ml}$$

$$62.5x = 500$$

$$x = 8\ ml$$

To administer 100 mg of drug, give 8 ml Dynapen.

17. a. For IM use add 3.5 ml diluent = 250 mg/ml.

    b.
$$\frac{0.75\ g}{250\ ml} = \frac{\overset{3}{\cancel{750\ mg}}}{\underset{1}{\cancel{250\ mg}}} \times 1\ ml$$

$$= 3\ ml$$

$$\frac{250\ mg}{1\ ml} :: \frac{750\ mg}{x\ ml}$$

$$250x = 750$$

$$x = 3\ ml$$

18. a. 18 ml   *OR*   8 ml

    b. 250,000 U/ml   *OR*   500,000 U/ml

    c. 5 million units

    d.
$$\frac{\overset{6}{\cancel{300,000\ U}}}{\underset{5}{\cancel{250,000\ U}}} \times 1\ ml = \frac{6}{5}$$

$$= 1.2\ ml$$

$$\frac{\overset{3}{\cancel{300,000\ U}}}{\underset{5}{\cancel{500,000\ U}}} \times 1\ ml = \frac{3}{5}$$

$$= 0.6\ ml$$

OR   *OR*

$$\frac{250,000\ U}{1\ ml} :: \frac{300,000\ U}{x\ ml}$$

$$250,000x = 300,000$$

$$x = 1.2\ ml$$

$$\frac{500,000\ U}{1\ ml} :: \frac{300,000\ U}{x\ ml}$$

$$500,000x = 300,000$$

$$x = 0.6\ ml$$

19. a. Add 1.8 ml diluent. Resulting solution contains 250 mg/ml.

b.

$$\frac{\overset{3}{\cancel{150}\ \text{mg}}}{\underset{5}{\cancel{250}\ \text{mg}}} \times 1\ \text{ml} = \frac{3}{5}$$

$$= 0.6\ \text{ml}$$

$$\frac{250\ \text{mg}}{1\ \text{ml}} :: \frac{150\ \text{mg}}{x\ \text{ml}}$$

$$250x = 150$$

$$x = 0.6\ \text{ml}$$

Add 0.6 ml ampicillin to the Buretrol.

$$\begin{array}{r} 100.0\ \text{ml solution} \\ -0.6\ \text{ml ampicillin} \\ \hline 99.4\ \text{ml D}_5\text{W} \end{array}$$

Add 99.4 ml D$_5$W to the Buretrol.

20.

$$\overset{25\ \text{ml/hr}}{4\ \text{hr})\overline{100\ \text{ml}}}$$

$$\frac{60\ \text{gtt/ml}}{60\ \text{min}} \times 25\ \text{ml} = 25\ \text{gtt/min the IV should infuse}$$

21. The IV should be running at 25 ml/hr, so 75 ml should have infused by 1500; it is 5 ml behind schedule.

$$25\ \text{ml} \times 3\ \text{hr} = 75\ \text{ml}$$

$$\frac{25\ \text{ml}}{1\ \text{hr}} :: \frac{x\ \text{ml}}{3\ \text{hr}}$$

$$x = 75\ \text{ml}$$

Because 1 hour remains and there is 30 ml left to infuse, we calculate the new flow rate as follows:

$$\frac{60\ \text{gtt/ml}}{60\ \text{min}} \times 30\ \text{ml} = 30\ \text{gtt/min the IV should infuse}$$

22.

$$\overset{12.25\ \text{ml/hr}}{4\ \text{hr})\overline{49.00\ \text{ml}}}$$
$$\begin{array}{r}4\\\hline 9\\8\\\hline 10\\8\\\hline 20\\20\end{array}$$

$$\frac{\dfrac{1}{\cancel{15}\text{ gtt/ml}}}{\dfrac{\cancel{60}\text{ min}}{4}} \times 12.25\text{ ml} = \frac{12.25}{4} = 3.06 \approx 3\text{ gtt/min}$$

$$\frac{\dfrac{1}{\cancel{60}\text{ gtt/ml}}}{\dfrac{\cancel{60}\text{ min}}{1}} \times 12.25\text{ ml} = 12.25 \approx 12\text{ gtt/min}$$

23.
$$10.2\text{ lb} \div 2.2\text{ lb/kg} = 4.636 \approx 4.64\text{ kg}$$

$$0.25\text{ mg/kg} \times 4.64\text{ kg} = 1.16\text{ mg}$$

$$1\text{ mg/kg} \times 4.64\text{ kg} = 4.64\text{ mg}$$

Yes, 4 mg falls within the manufacturer's recommended dosage range.

24.
$$\frac{\dfrac{2}{\cancel{60}\text{ gtt/ml}}}{\dfrac{\cancel{30}\text{ min}}{1}} \times 50\text{ ml} = 100\text{ gtt/min}$$

25. First convert the 4 oz to pounds: if 16 oz = 1 lb, then 4 oz = ¼ lb, or 0.25 lb.

$$13.25\text{ lb} \div 2.2\text{ lb/kg} = 6.023 \approx 6.02\text{ kg}$$

$$7.5\text{ mg/kg} \times 6.02\text{ kg} = 45.15\text{ mg}$$

$$45.15 \div 3 = 15.05\text{ mg/dose}$$

The doctor's order is less than the recommended 15.05 mg/dose; only 12.5 mg was ordered. Question this order.

26. a.
$$143\text{ lb} \div 2.2\text{ lb/kg} = 65\text{ kg}$$
$$0.025\text{ ml/kg/min} \times 65\text{ kg} = 1.625\text{ ml/min}$$

   b.
$$1.625\text{ ml/min} \times 60\text{ gtt/ml} = 97.5 \approx 98\text{ gtt/min}$$

   c.
$$1.625\text{ ml/min} \times 20\text{ gtt/ml} = 32.5 \approx 33\text{ gtt/min}$$

27. a. 11 lb   =   <u>0.29</u> m^2

   b. 26 lb   =   <u>0.535</u> m^2

   c. 62.5 lb =   <u>1.00</u> m^2

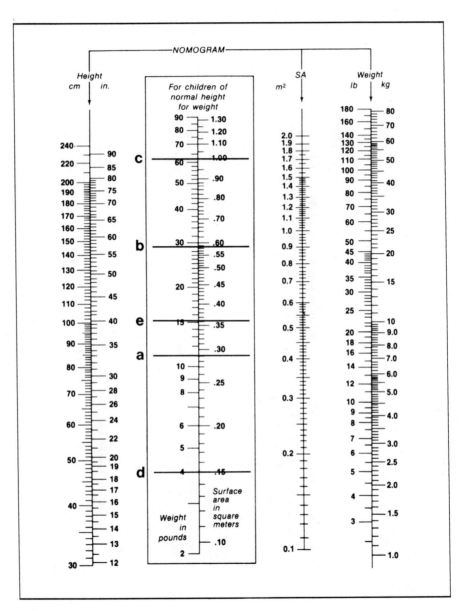

Answers: BSA (m²) for problem 27.

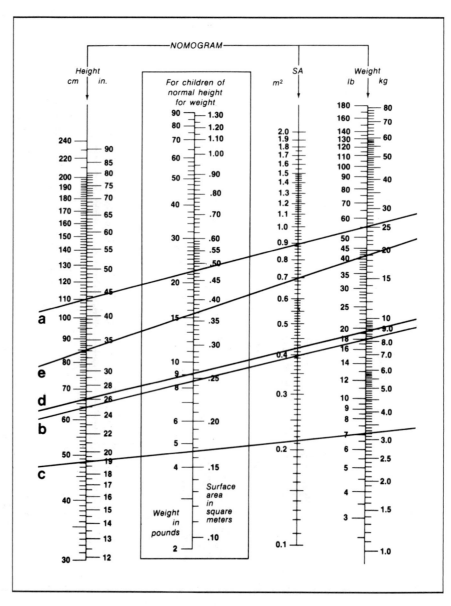

—NOMOGRAM—

Answers: BSA (m²) for problem 28.

d. 4 lb   =   <u>   0.15   </u>   m²

e. 15 lb   =   <u>   0.36   </u>   m²

See nomogram, page 273.

28. a. 0.88 m²

   b. 0.4 m²

   c. 0.22 m²

   d. 0.42 m²

   e. 0.7 m²

See nomogram, page 274.

29.
$$\frac{BSA\ (m^2) \times adult\ dose}{1.7\ m^2} = Child's\ dose$$

$$\frac{0.22\ m^2 \times 75\ mg}{1.7\ m^2} = \frac{16.5}{1.7} = 9.7\ mg$$

30.
$$60\ mg/m^2 \times 1.2\ m^2 = 72\ mg$$
$$250\ mg/m^2 \times 1.2\ m^2 = 300\ mg$$

Dosage range is 72 to 300 mg/dose.

PRACTICE TEST 4

Read all problems carefully. Work accurately. Label each answer.

1. The physician orders 0.375 mg digoxin.
   The tablets on hand are 0.25 mg strength.
   Give _____

2. The physician orders Thiosulfil 1 g.
   The tablets on hand are 250 mg.
   Give _____

3. Convert the following temperatures:
   a. 50 °F = _____ °C
   b. 72 °C = _____ °F

4. The physician orders 10 g chloral hydrate. Available is a vial containing a 25 percent solution.
   Give _____

5. The physician orders 3000 ml D₅RL to be given in 24 hours. The drop factor is 20 gtt/ml. At what flow rate (gtt/min) should this IV be set?

6. The physician orders liver extract 80 mcg.
   The vial available is labeled 200 mcg per 10 ml.
   Give _____

7. The physician orders calcium gluceptate 540 mg to be added to IV fluids. You have available 5-ml ampules containing 90 mg calcium gluceptate.
   Add _____

8. You must give potassium chloride 40 mEq. You have a unit dose bottle containing 20 mEq per 10 ml.
   Give _____

9. You must give Polycillin 1 g po. You have available a 100-ml bottle of Polycillin for oral suspension. To prepare it is necessary to add a total of 81 ml water and shake well. This provides 100 ml of suspension. Each 5 ml contains Polycillin equivalent to 250 mg.
   Give _____

10. The physician orders 15,000 U heparin. The vial on hand is labeled heparin 20,000 U/ml.
Give _____

11. The order is for penicillin 1,500,000 U from a solution labeled 3,000,000 U per 5 ml.
Give _____

12. The order is for Dilaudid gr ⅙. On hand are gr ⅓ tablets.
Give _____

13. The order is for atropine sulfate gr ¹⁄₂₀₀. The available tablets are gr ¹⁄₃₀₀.
Give _____

14. How will you make 1 L of 35 percent cresol solution? Cresol is a pure liquid drug.
Drug _____
Solvent _____

15. Prepare 250 ml physiologic salt solution (0.9 percent) using salt crystals.
Drug _____
Solvent _____

16. The adult dose is 300,000 U penicillin. Using Clark's rule, how much penicillin will a 50-lb child receive? _____

17. Using Clark's rule, what is the average dose for a child weighing 60 lb if an adult dose of Terramycin is 100 mg? _____

18. How would you prepare 85 U of U100 NPH insulin using an insulin syringe? Using a tuberculin syringe?

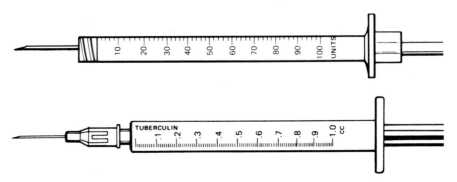

19. 15 gr _____ g
    4 dr _____ oz
    1 qt _____ ml
    ½ oz _____ Tbs
    4000 ml _____ gal

20. 1 ml _____ minims
    1 pt (O i) _____ ml
    1 tsp _____ ℥ _____ ml
    30 ml _____ Tbs

21. Give 400,000 U potassium penicillin G.

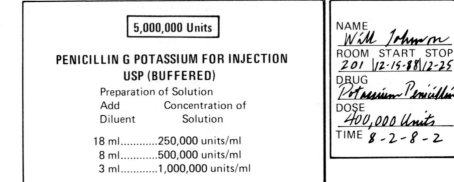

5,000,000 Units

PENICILLIN G POTASSIUM FOR INJECTION
USP (BUFFERED)

Preparation of Solution

Add Diluent	Concentration of Solution
18 ml	250,000 units/ml
8 ml	500,000 units/ml
3 ml	1,000,000 units/ml

NAME *Will Johnson*
ROOM START STOP
201 *12-15-88*|*12-25*
DRUG *Potassium Penicillin*
DOSE *400,000 Units*
TIME *8 - 2 - 8 - 2*

   a. How much diluent must you add to make the strength
      needed? _____

   b. What is the dosage strength of the solution you mixed? _____

   c. How much potassium penicillin G does this vial contain? _____

   d. Compute dosage to be given.

22. Use Freid's rule to determine the dosage for an 11-month-old infant for a drug when the adult dose is 240 mg.

23. Use Young's rule to determine the safe dose of a medication for a 7-year-old child when the adult dose is 30 mg.

24. The recommended dose of streptomycin for a premature infant is 15 to 30 mg/kg/day. What is the recommended dosage range for a 4-lb infant?

25. Use the West nomogram (page 265) determine the BSA for a child weighing 33 lb with a height of 34 inches. Use the BSA formula to calculate the dosage of a drug if the adult dose is 75 mg.

26. Look at the computer printout sheet (page 230). State in traditional time the hours Mr. Apple is to receive Terbutaline.

27. An intravenous medication has been reconstituted into 60 ml of solution. The medication is to be administered in 30 minutes. The drop factor is 20 gtt/ml. At what flow rate (gtt/min) should this IV infuse?

28. The physician ordered 20 g $MgSO_4$ to be added to 1000 ml D_5W, and

infuse at 1.5 g/hr. The drop factor is 13 gtt/ml. How much fluid is to be infused in 1 hour? At what flow rate (gtt/min) should this IV infuse?

29. Prepare 500 ml of a 0.5 percent solution from a 2 percent solution.
Solute _____
Solvent _____

30. If 375 ml of drug is used to prepare 1500 ml solution, what is the percentage strength of this solution?

31. Convert
    65 lb = _____ kg
    225 lb = _____ kg
    75 kg = _____ lb
    33 kg = _____ lb
    3.8 kg = _____ lb

32. 2325   = _____ Regular time
    0630   = _____ Regular time
    1606   = _____ Regular time
    4:45 AM = _____ 24-hour clock
    9:30 PM = _____ 24-hour clock
    12:15 AM = _____ 24-hour clock

ANSWERS: PRACTICE TEST 4

1. $\dfrac{0.375 \text{ mg}}{0.25 \text{ mg}} \times 1 \text{ tab} = 1\dfrac{1}{2} \text{ tab}$ $\dfrac{0.25 \text{ mg}}{1 \text{ tab}} :: \dfrac{0.375}{x \text{ tab}}$

$$0.25x = 0.375$$

$$x = 1.5 \text{ or } 1\frac{1}{2} \text{ tab}$$

Give 1½ tablets of digoxin 0.25 mg.

2. 1 g = 1000 mg

$$\frac{\overset{4}{\cancel{1000}} \text{ mg}}{\underset{1}{\cancel{250}} \text{ mg}} \times 1 \text{ tab} = 4 \text{ tab}$$

$$\frac{250 \text{ mg}}{1 \text{ tab}} :: \frac{1000 \text{ mg}}{x \text{ tab}}$$

$$250x = 1000$$

$$x = 4 \text{ tab}$$

Give 4 tablets of 250 mg Thiosulfil.

3. a.

$$1.8 \,°C = F - 32$$

$$1.8 \,°C = 50 - 32$$

$$1.8 \,°C = 18$$

$$\frac{1.8}{1.8} \,°C = \frac{18}{1.8}$$

$$°C = 10$$

$$°C = (F - 32) \times \frac{5}{9}$$

$$°C = (50 - 32) \times \frac{5}{9}$$

$$°C = 18 \times \frac{5}{9}$$

$$°C = \frac{90}{9}$$

$$°C = 10$$

   b.

$$1.8 \,°C = °F - 32$$

$$1.8 \times 72 = °F - 32$$

$$32 + 129.6 = °F - 32 + 32$$

$$161.6 = °F$$

$$°F = \left(\frac{9}{5} \,°C\right) + 32$$

$$°F = \left(\frac{9}{5} \times 72\right) + 32$$

$$°F = \left(\frac{648}{5}\right) + 32$$

$$°F = 129.6 + 32$$

$$°F = 161.6$$

4.

$$\frac{10 \text{ g}}{25 \text{ g}} \times 100 \text{ ml} = 40 \text{ ml}$$

$$\frac{25 \text{ g}}{100 \text{ ml}} :: \frac{10 \text{ g}}{x \text{ ml}}$$

$$25x = 1000$$

$$x = 40$$

Give 40 ml chloral hydrate.

5.

$$125 \text{ ml} = 1\text{-hr volume}$$

$$24\overline{)3000} \text{ ml} = 24\text{-hr volume}$$

$$
\begin{array}{r}
\underline{24} \\
60 \\
\underline{48} \\
120 \\
\underline{120} \\
0
\end{array}
$$

$$\frac{20 \text{ gtt/ml}}{60 \text{ min}} \times 125 \text{ ml} = \frac{125}{3} \approx 42 \text{ gtt/min}$$

Run IV at 42 gtt/min.

6.

$$\frac{\overset{8}{\cancel{80} \text{ mcg}}}{\underset{\underset{2}{\cancel{20}}}{\cancel{200} \text{ mcg}}} \times \overset{1}{\cancel{10} \text{ ml}} = \frac{8}{2}$$

$$= 4 \text{ ml}$$

$$\frac{200 \text{ mcg}}{10 \text{ ml}} :: \frac{80 \text{ mcg}}{x \text{ ml}}$$

$$200x = 800$$

$$x = 4 \text{ ml}$$

Give 4 ml liver extract.

7.

$$\frac{\overset{6}{\cancel{540} \text{ mg}}}{\underset{1}{\cancel{90} \text{ mg}}} \times 5 \text{ ml} = 30 \text{ ml}$$

$$\frac{90 \text{ mg}}{5 \text{ ml}} :: \frac{540 \text{ mg}}{x \text{ ml}}$$

$$90x = 2700$$

$$x = 30 \text{ ml}$$

Give 30 ml calcium gluceptate. As it comes in 5-ml ampules, you will need to use 6 ampules.

8.

$$\frac{\overset{2}{\cancel{40} \text{ mEq}}}{\underset{1}{\cancel{20} \text{ mEq}}} \times 10 \text{ ml} = 20 \text{ ml}$$

$$\frac{20 \text{ mEq}}{10 \text{ ml}} :: \frac{40 \text{ mEq}}{x \text{ ml}}$$

$$20x = 400$$

$$x = 20 \text{ ml}$$

Give 20 ml potassium chloride.

9.

$$\dfrac{\overset{4}{\cancel{1000}\text{ mg}}}{\underset{1}{\cancel{250}\text{ mg}}} \times 5 \text{ ml} = 20 \text{ ml}$$

$$\dfrac{250 \text{ mg}}{5 \text{ ml}} :: \dfrac{1000 \text{ mg}}{x \text{ ml}}$$

$$250x = 5000$$

$$x = 20 \text{ ml}$$

Give 20 ml Polycillin.

10.

$$\dfrac{\overset{3}{\cancel{15,000}\text{ U}}}{\underset{4}{\cancel{20,000}\text{ U}}} \times 1 \text{ ml} = \dfrac{3}{4}$$

$$= 0.75 \text{ ml}$$

$$\dfrac{20,000 \text{ U}}{1 \text{ ml}} :: \dfrac{15,000 \text{ U}}{x \text{ ml}}$$

$$20,000x = 15,000$$

$$x = 0.75 \text{ ml}$$

Give 0.75 ml heparin.

11.

$$\dfrac{\overset{1}{\cancel{1,500,000}\text{ U}}}{\underset{2}{\cancel{3,000,000}\text{ U}}} \times 5 \text{ ml} = \dfrac{5}{2}$$

$$= 2.5 \text{ ml}$$

$$\dfrac{3,000,000 \text{ U}}{5 \text{ ml}} :: \dfrac{1,500,000 \text{ U}}{x \text{ ml}}$$

$$3,000,000x = 7,500,000$$

$$x = 2.5 \text{ ml}$$

Give 2.5 ml penicillin.

12.

$$\dfrac{\frac{1}{6}\text{ gr}}{\frac{1}{3}\text{ gr}} \times 1 \text{ tab} = x$$

$$\dfrac{1}{6} \div \dfrac{1}{3} \times 1 = x$$

$$\dfrac{1}{\cancel{6}} \times \dfrac{\overset{1}{\cancel{3}}}{1} \times 1 = \dfrac{1}{2} \text{ tab}$$

$$\dfrac{\frac{1}{3}\text{ gr}}{1 \text{ tab}} :: \dfrac{\frac{1}{6}\text{ gr}}{x \text{ tab}}$$

$$\dfrac{1}{3}x = \dfrac{1}{6}$$

$$x = \dfrac{1}{6} \div \dfrac{1}{3}$$

$$x = \dfrac{1}{\cancel{6}} \times \dfrac{\overset{1}{\cancel{3}}}{1}$$

$$x = \dfrac{1}{2} \text{ tab}$$

Give ½ tablet of Dilaudid gr ⅓.

13.

$$\frac{gr \dfrac{1}{200}}{gr \dfrac{1}{300}} \times 1 \text{ tab} = x$$

$$\frac{1}{200} \div \frac{1}{300} \times 1 = x$$

$$\frac{1}{\underset{2}{\cancel{200}}} \times \frac{\cancel{300}}{1} \times 1 = \frac{3}{2}$$

$$= 1\frac{1}{2} \text{ tab}$$

$$\frac{gr \dfrac{1}{300}}{1 \text{ tab}} :: \frac{gr \dfrac{1}{200}}{x \text{ tab}}$$

$$\frac{1}{300} x = \frac{1}{200}$$

$$x = \frac{1}{200} \div \frac{1}{300}$$

$$x = \frac{1}{200} \times \frac{300}{1}$$

$$x = 1\frac{1}{2} \text{ tab}$$

Give 1½ tablets of atropine sulfate.

14.

$$\frac{35 \text{ ml}}{\underset{1}{\cancel{100} \text{ ml}}} \times \overset{10}{\cancel{1000}} \text{ ml} = 350 \text{ ml}$$

$$\frac{35 \text{ ml}}{100 \text{ ml}} :: \frac{x \text{ ml}}{1000 \text{ ml}}$$

$$100x = 35,000$$

$$x = 350 \text{ ml}$$

$$1000 \text{ ml solution}$$
$$\underline{- 350 \text{ ml cresol}}$$
$$650 \text{ ml solvent}$$

15.

$$\frac{0.9 \text{ g}}{\underset{2}{\cancel{100} \text{ ml}}} \times \overset{5}{\cancel{250}} \text{ ml} = \frac{4.5}{2}$$

$$= 2.25 \text{ g}$$

$$\frac{0.9 \text{ g}}{100 \text{ ml}} :: \frac{x \text{ g}}{250 \text{ ml}}$$

$$100x = 225$$

$$x = 2.25 \text{ g}$$

The solute is 2.25 g salt. For the solvent, place 2.25 g salt crystals in a container and add enough water to equal 250 ml.

16.

$$\frac{50 \text{ lb}}{\underset{1}{\cancel{150} \text{ lb}}} \times \overset{2000}{\cancel{300,000}} \text{ U} = 100,000 \text{ U penicillin}$$

17.

$$\frac{\overset{20}{\cancel{60} \text{ lb}}}{\underset{3}{\cancel{150} \text{ lb}}} \times \overset{2}{\cancel{100}} \text{ mg} = 40 \text{ mg Terramycin}$$

18. Using a U100 insulin syringe, draw up Lente U100 insulin to the 85U mark on the syringe.

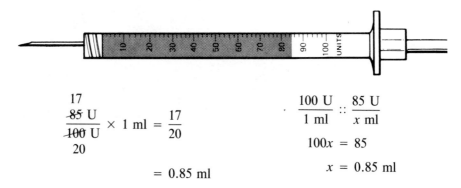

$$\dfrac{\overset{17}{\cancel{85\ U}}}{\underset{20}{\cancel{100\ U}}} \times 1\ ml = \dfrac{17}{20}$$

$$= 0.85\ ml$$

$$\dfrac{100\ U}{1\ ml} :: \dfrac{85\ U}{x\ ml}$$

$$100x = 85$$

$$x = 0.85\ ml$$

Give 0.85 ml Lente U100 insulin in a tuberculin syringe.

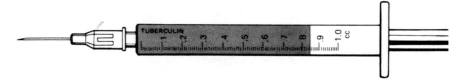

19. 5 gr = 1 g
    4 dr = ½ oz
    1 qt = 1000 ml
    ½ oz = 1 Tbs
    4000 ml = 1 gal

20. 1 ml = 15 minims
    1 pt = 500 ml
    1 tsp = ℨ i or 4 to 5 ml
    30 ml = 2 Tbs

21. a. 8 ml diluent

    b. 500,000 U/ml = dosage strength

    c. 5,000,000 U = contents of the bottle

    d. $$\dfrac{\overset{4}{\cancel{400,000\ U}}}{\underset{5}{\cancel{500,000\ U}}} \times 1\ ml = \dfrac{4}{5}$$

    $$= 0.8\ ml$$

    $$\dfrac{500,000\ U}{1\ ml} :: \dfrac{400,000\ U}{x\ ml}$$

    $$500,000x = 400,000$$

    $$x = 0.8\ ml$$

Give 0.8 ml penicillin.

22.
$$\frac{\text{Age of infant in months}}{150 \text{ lb}} \times \text{adult dose} = \text{Child's dose}$$

$$\frac{11 \text{ months}}{\underset{15}{\cancel{150} \text{ lb}}} \times \overset{24}{\cancel{240}} \text{ mg} = \frac{264}{15}$$

$$= 17.6 \text{ mg}$$

23.
$$\frac{\text{Age of child in years}}{\text{Age of child in years} + 12} \times \text{adult dose} = \text{Child's dose}$$

$$\frac{7 \text{ yr}}{7 \text{ yr} + 12} \times 30 \text{ mg} = \frac{7}{19} \times 30$$

$$= \frac{210}{19}$$

$$= 11.05 \text{ mg}$$

24.
$$4 \text{ lb} \div 2.2 \text{ lb/kg} = 1.818 \text{ kg}$$

$$15 \text{ mg/kg/day} \times 1.818 \text{ kg} = 27.27 \text{ mg/day}$$

$$30 \text{ mg/kg/day} \times 1.818 \text{ kg} = 54.54 \text{ mg/day}$$

The dosage range of streptomycin for a 4-lb infant is 27.27 to 54.54 mg/day.

25. BSA $= 0.61 \text{ m}^2$

$$\frac{\text{BSA (m}^2)}{1.7 \text{ m}^2} \times \text{adult dose} = \text{Child's dose}$$

$$\frac{0.61 \text{ m}^2}{1.7 \text{ m}^2} \times 75 \text{ mg} = \frac{45.75}{1.7}$$

$$= 26.911$$

$$\approx 26.91 \text{ mg}$$

26. 10 AM, 4 PM, and 10 PM

27.
$$\frac{\underset{\underset{1}{\cancel{3}}}{\cancel{20} \text{ gtt/ml}}}{\cancel{30} \text{ min}} \times \overset{20}{\cancel{60}} \text{ ml} = 40 \text{ gtt/min IV should infuse}$$

28.
$$\frac{1.5 \text{ g/hr}}{\underset{1}{\cancel{20} \text{ g}}} \times \cancel{1000}^{\,50} \text{ ml} = 75 \text{ ml/hr}$$

$$\frac{20 \text{ g}}{1000 \text{ ml}} :: \frac{1.5 \text{ g/hr}}{x \text{ ml}}$$

$$20x = 1500$$

$$x = 75 \text{ ml/hr}$$

Infuse $MgSO_4$ at 75 ml/hr to administer 1.5 g $MgSO_4$.

$$\frac{13 \text{ gtt/ml}}{\underset{12}{\cancel{60} \text{ min}}} \times \cancel{75}^{\,15} \text{ ml} = \frac{195}{12}$$

$$= 16.25$$

$$\approx 16 \text{ gtt/min IV should infuse}$$

29.
$$\frac{0.5 \text{ ml}}{2 \text{ ml}} \times 500 \text{ ml} = 125 \text{ ml}$$

$$\frac{2 \text{ ml}}{500 \text{ ml}} :: \frac{0.5 \text{ ml}}{x \text{ ml}}$$

$$2x = 250.0$$

$$x = 125 \text{ ml}$$

You need 125 ml of the 2 percent solution to make 500 ml of a 0.5 percent solution.

$$\begin{array}{r} 500 \text{ ml solution} \\ - 125 \text{ ml 2 percent solution (solute)} \\ \hline 375 \text{ ml solvent needed} \end{array}$$

30.
$$\frac{x \text{ ml}}{\underset{1}{\cancel{100} \text{ ml}}} \times \cancel{1500}^{\,15} \text{ ml} = 375 \text{ ml}$$

$$\frac{x \text{ ml}}{100 \text{ ml}} :: \frac{375 \text{ ml}}{1500 \text{ ml}}$$

$$1500x = 37,500$$

$$x = 25 \text{ ml}$$

$$15x = 375$$

$$x = 25 \text{ ml}$$

$$\frac{25}{100} = 25 \text{ percent solution}$$

31. 65 lb = 29.545 ≈ 29.55 kg
    225 lb = 102.272 ≈ 102.27 kg
    75 kg = 165 lb
    33 kg = 72.6 lb
    3.8 kg = 8.36 lb

32. 2325   =   <u>11:25 PM</u>   Regular time

    0630   =   <u>6:30 AM</u>   Regular time

    1606   =   <u>4:06 PM</u>   Regular time

    4:45 AM   =   <u>0445</u>   24-hour clock

    9:30 PM   =   <u>2130</u>   24-hour clock

    12:15 AM   =   <u>0015</u>   24-hour clock